Manual of SQUINT

AF693530

Manual of SQUINT

Leela Ahuja
Ex-Professor of Strabismology
Ex-Director, Institute of Ophthalmology
Aligarh Muslim University
Aligarh, UP
India

JAYPEE

JAYPEE BROTHERS MEDICAL PUBLISHERS
The Health Sciences Publisher
New Delhi | London

Jaypee Brothers Medical Publishers (P) Ltd

Headquarters
EMCA House, 23/23-B Ansari Road,
Daryaganj New Delhi 110 002, India
Landline: +91-11-23272143,
+91-11-23272703
+91-11-23282021, +91-11-23245672
e-mail: jaypee@jaypeebrothers.com

Corporate Office
4838/24, Ansari Road,
Daryaganj New Delhi 110 002, India
Phone: +91-11-43574357
Fax: +91-11-43574314
e-mail: jaypee@jaypeebrothers.com

Overseas Office
JP Medical Ltd.
83, Victoria Street, London
SW1H 0HW (UK)
Phone: +44-20 3170 8910
e-mail: info@jpmedpub.com

EU GPSR Authorised Representative
Logos Europe, 9 rue Nicolas Poussin
17000, La Rochelle, France
Phone: +33 (0) 6 67 93 73 78
e-mail: contact@logoseurope.eu

Website: www.jaypeebrothers.com
Website: www.jaypeedigital.com
© 2008, Jaypee Brothers Medical Publishers
All brand names and product names used in this book are trade names, service marks, trademarks or registered trademarks of their respective owners. The publisher is not associated with any product or vendor mentioned in this book.
Medical knowledge and practice change constantly. This book is designed to provide accurate, authoritative information about the subject matter in question. However, readers are advised to check the most current information available on procedures included and check information from the manufacturer of each product to be administered, to verify the recommended dose, formula, method and duration of administration, adverse effects and contraindications. It is the responsibility of the practitioner to take all appropriate safety precautions. Neither the publisher nor the author(s)/editor(s) assume any liability for any injury and/or damage to persons or property arising from or related to use of material in this book.
This book is sold on the understanding that the publisher is not engaged in providing professional medical services. If such advice or services are required, the services of a competent medical professional should be sought.
Every effort has been made where necessary to contact holders of copyright to obtain permission to reproduce copyright material. If any have been inadvertently overlooked, the publisher will be pleased to make the necessary arrangements at the first opportunity.
Inquiries for bulk sales may be solicited at: jaypee@jaypeebrothers.com

Manual of Squint

First Edition: 2008
Reprint: **2026**
ISBN 978-81-8448-382-6

Printed in India

To

— Shridivale Sai Baba

— My Husband Prof. (Dr) OP Ahuja
Ex-Director of Institute of Ophthalmology and Director, Founder of Ahuja Eye Centre, Aligarh

— My grandchildren– Ashir, Arjun, Shishir, Aanchal, Rhea and Savani — the future of India

Preface

A lot of literary works have been done on squint but still there is a dearth of standard books on strabismus for postgraduate students. No doubt, surgery of squint is done by many ophthalmologists, but mostly, it is on cosmetic grounds and that too without the help of proper orthoptic department. It is also a fact that general public is reluctant to have treatment, particularly surgical treatment of squint, as this malady is considered to be due to displeasure of some Goddess. The importance is not to cure deviation, but to improve binocular function. Blindness has existed since time immemorial as illustrated in the story of Shravan Kumar.

I realize that some of the topics are very much comprehensive so I have tried to simplify them by providing their description in simple and easily understood language. Most controversial aspects of certain conditions have been deliberately left out for the sake of easy understanding. This book includes material from Duke-Elder, Kyth Lyle, von Noordan, Kanski, Muller and Paymann. The first three chapters on applied anatomy of paralytic squint are venture of my husband Prof OP Ahuja, Ex-Director, Institute of Ophthalmology, and Founder and Director of Ahuja Eye Centre, Aligarh, UP.

I owe so much to Prof GP Gupta, Ex-Director of Institute of Ophthalmology, Aligarh, Prof BS Goel, Ex-Director, Institute of Ophthalmology, Aligarh and my son Dr Anupam Ahuja, Consultant, Ahuja Eye Centre, Aligarh for help and providing me photographs.

I am immensely thankful to Late (Prof) LP Agarwal, Ex-Director AIIMS, Delhi, Prof (Dr) Manoj Shukla, Ex-Director, Institute of Ophthalmology, Aligarh, Prof (Dr) SS Soodan, Principal and Director of Ascon College of Medical Science, Jammu, Prof S Mittal, Head, Department of Ophthalmology, Meerut Medical College, Prof BD Sharma, Head, Department of Ophthalmology, Agra Medical College, Prof RC Nagpal, Head, Dept. of Ophthalmology, Jolly Grant Medical College, Dehradun and Dr Bhavna Chawla, Assistant Professor, Department of Ophthalmology, AIIMS, New Delhi for their support.

Moreover, I would like to thank Dr Namrata Bhardwaj, Dr Awadesh Bhardwaj, Dr Gyatri Ahuja, Dr Indira Mehrotra, Dr Naintara Vasudeva, Dr Sheela Sachdeva, Dr Usha Chawla, Dr Shashi Ahuja, Mrs Vimal Narula, Mrs Manju Ahuja and Mrs Aruna Ahuja for their encouragement to me.

My sincere thanks to Mr Zaheer Ahmad (Limra Computers), Rumana Naz (Artist) and Mr Kanaihya (Typist) for help.

I am extremely grateful to Aligarh Muslim University for giving me opportunity to serve in the Department of Ophthalmology for 33 years.

My special thanks to my publisher Shri JP Vij, CEO, editorial board and the other staff of M/s Jaypee Brothers Medical Publishers (P) Ltd., New Delhi for giving me this opportunity to author this book.

Last, but not the least, the strength and energy given by God alone could have made me complete this book.

Leela Ahuja

Contents

1 Introduction

The strabismus, a condition of lack of coordination between the two eyes is known and recognized since the earliest time. In the primitive folklore and mythology, it was considered to be an effect of evil eye. The word strabismus was derived from the name of Greek Geographer named, 'STRABO' who had a horrible and unbecoming squint. The reorganistic and documentation of the condition of the squint in the literature dated back to 2600 BC. It was stated that Egyptian Goddess Maya Squinted and also Egyptian King D Joser (2600 BC) for whom the first pyramid was built, has gross internal squint, Guillemean described strabismus as a wrestling or within which drawth the sight unequally or a convulsion and pulling of muscles which move the eye or so same muscles of the eye are loosened and shortened, so the eyes as drawn downward, upward, to the right side or to the left side.

Hippocrates first noted the cross eye in children of cross eyes parents use of a mask with two holes in front of the eyes to straighten them was described by Paulus, Worth in 1903 classified the binocular vision in three grades and devised the four dot test. Maddox emphasized the treatment of abnormal retinal correspondence and Mary Maddox was first to organize the orthoptic clinic in London.

The prevalence of squint in Indian population to be 3-4% and prevalence of amblyopia 1%.

2 Anatomy of Extraocular Muscles

The eyeball is moved by a set of six extraocular muscles, consisting of four recti and two oblique muscles. These arise from the wall of the orbit, and are inserted into the sclera.

The four recti (medial, lateral, superior and inferior) arise from the circumference of the optic foramen at the apex of the orbit, run forward, surrounding the optic nerve and posterior part of the eyeball, and are inserted into the sclera by means of flattened tendons, about 10 mm wide **(Table 2.1)**.

TABLE 2.1: Showing the measurements of the tendons of recti muscles and the distance of their insertion from the limbus

Muscle	*Distance of insertion from the limbus (mm)*	*Length of tendon (mm)*	*Width of tendon (mm)*
Medial rectus	5.5	3.7	10.3
Inferior rectus	6.5	5.5	9.8
Lateral rectus	6.9	8.8	9.2
Superior rectus	7.7	5.0	10.6

As evident from the table, the lines of insertion of these muscles are not equidistant from the limbus, but are somewhat in the form of spiral (Spiral of Tillaux) **(Fig. 2.1)** superior rectus and medial rectus are closely attached to the dural sheath of optic nerve, at their origin. This accounts for the characteristic pain felt on moving the eyeball up and in, in a case of retrobulbar neuritis.

The superior oblique arises from the bone at the upper and inner border of the optic foramen, and runs forward to the upper and inner angle of the orbit, at the anterior extremity of which it passes through a fibrous pulley **(Fig. 2.2)**. It then continues backward and outward, passing beneath the superior rectus getting inserted to the upper and outer part of the sclera behind the equator **(Fig. 2.3)**. The inferior oblique arises

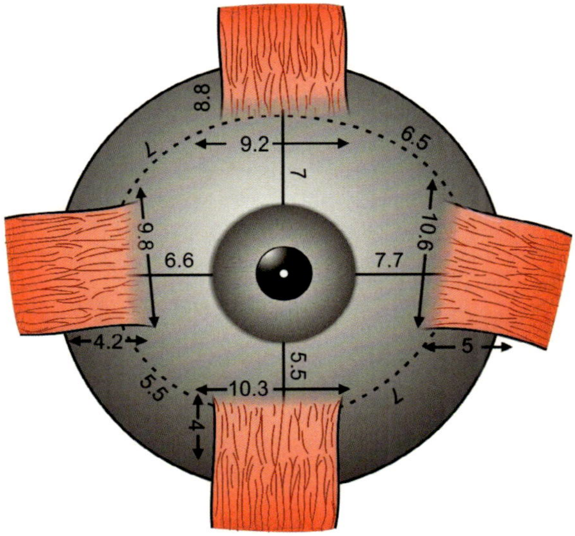

FIG. 2.1: Spiral of Tillaux

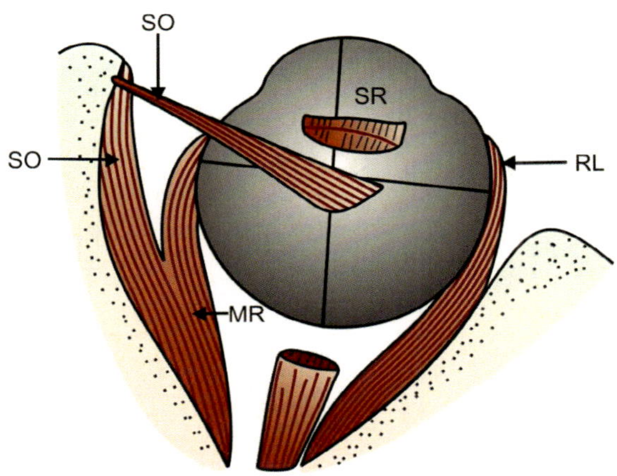

FIG. 2.2: Relation of insertion, superior muscles to the center of rotation of the eye

from the inner aspect of the superior maxillary bone at the lower border of orbit. It passes outwards below the inferior rectus and gets inserted into the outer part of the sclera behind the equator.

The long axis of the superior and inferior rectus (i.e. from its origin to the insertion) lies at an angle of 23° to the long axis of the eyeball. Likewise the axis of the superior and inferior oblique muscles make an

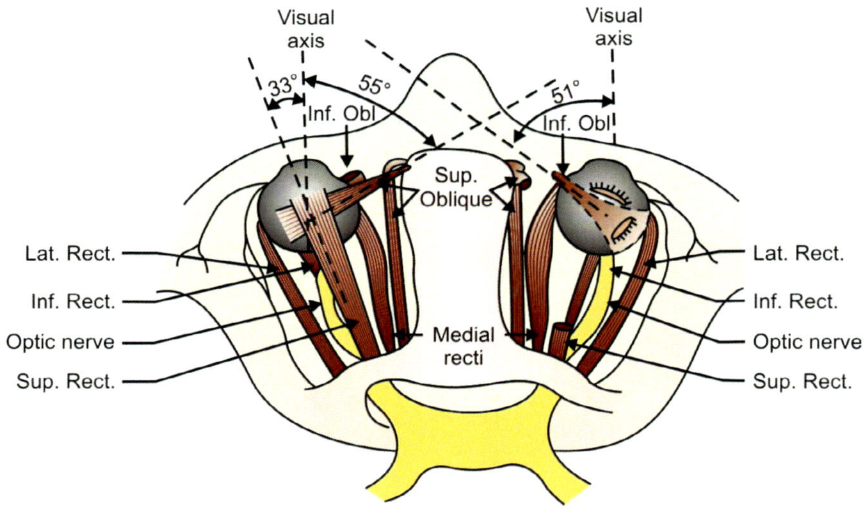

FIG. 2.3: Position of extrinsic ocular muscles

angle of 51° with the eyeball axis. These features are primarily responsible for determining the action of these muscles when the eyeball is turned from one particular position to the other.

The muscles are enclosed in a sheath derived from the fascia of the orbit, which covers the sclera as Tenon's capsule, and sends off prolongations to the walls of the orbit. Such prolongations are most prominent upon the medial and lateral rectus muscles. Termed as check ligaments **(Fig. 2.4),** they serve to restrain the excursions of the eyeball.

NERVE SUPPLY

The extrinsic muscles of the eye are supplied by the III, IV, and the VI cranial nerves.

The third or oculomotor nerve supplies the superior rectus (along with the levator muscle of the upper lid) through its superior division; and inferior rectus, medial rectus and inferior oblique muscles via its inferior division. The IIIN along with the IVN nucleus form a large mass of cells lying near the midline in the floor of the aqueduct of Sylvius beneath the superior colliculus. The cells nearest the midline in the anterior part are smaller and constitute the Edinger-Westphal nucleus which supplies the ciliary muscles (accommodation) and sphincter muscle (pupillary constriction). The main mass of the larger cells is further divided into cell masses serving the individual muscles. There is a considerable amount of decussation of fibers, particularly in the posterior part of the nucleus.

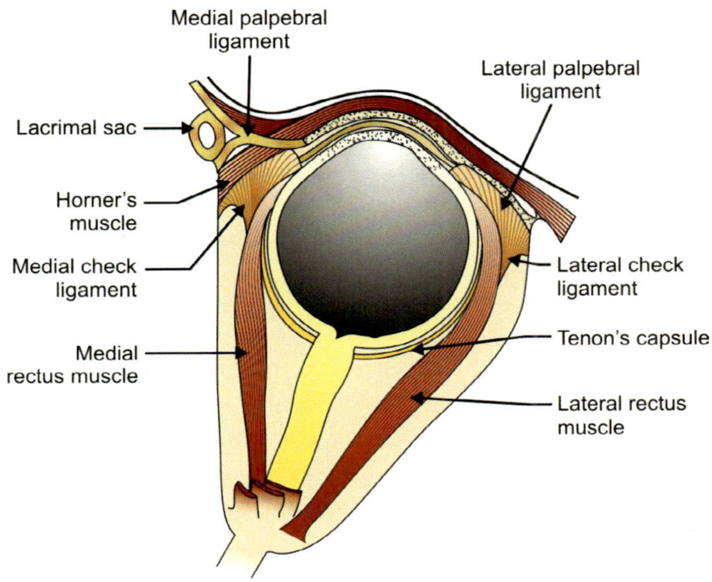

FIG. 2.4: Cleck ligaments

The fourth or the trochlear nerve supplies the superior oblique muscle. It is unique amongst the motor nerves that its fibers decussate dorsally, and are distributed to the superior oblique of the opposite side. The intracranial course of the fourth nerve is the longest of all the oculomotor nerves, its nucleus lies in the floor of the aqueduct of Sylvius overlapping the subnucleus of the inferior rectus muscle.

The sixth or the abducens nerve supplies the lateral rectus muscle. The intracranial course of the nerve is long, and all the fibers are distributed to the ipsilateral lateral rectus. Its nucleus lies in the floor of the fourth ventricle in the immediate vicinity of the seventh (Facial) nerve nucleus, the fibers from which make a large bend around it. Thus, vascular and other lesions of the VI nucleus are likely to accompany a facial paralysis on the same side.

3 *Neurological Control of Ocular Movements*

The action of III, IV and VI nerve is controlled and coordinated by a complex intermediary complex and 'centers' lying in the region of midbrain. The nuclei are interconnected to a considerable extent by fibers participating the posterior longitudinal bundle. These fibers play an important role in the coordination of ocular movements and equilibration. One of the most important of such connections is the link between the VI nerve nucleus of one side with the III nerve nucleus of the other. In this region there are also 'centers' that control the conjugate movements.

This elaborate mechanism in the midbrain is, in turn, controlled from three sources, one voluntary and three reflex.

Voluntary ocular movements. These are initiated in the motor area of frontal lobe of both sides. The fibers travel along the internal capsule, leaving it in the midbrain first the fibers for vertical movements and movements of the upper lid and then those for lateral movements. These fibers control the conjugate movement of both eyes, but movements of individual muscles are not represented. Stimulation of cortex or the tract therefore produces a conjugate deviation of eyes in the opposite direction, while a destruction would lead to a paralysis of conjugate movements away from affected side.

Psychoptic reflexes like fixation, fusional movements and convergence, etc. are centered in the visual cortex of occipital lobe. The afferent pathway is through the visual pathways, and the efferent run down the optic radiations to the posterior longitudinal bundle and then the oculomotor nerves.

Statokinetic reflex controls the position of eyes when the head is rotated in space. The afferent fibers run from the semicircular canals of the inner ears to the midbrain centers.

Static reflexes coordinate movements of eyes in respect of movement of the head on the body. These are initiated by the proprioceptive impulses arising from the neck muscles which are linked to the oculomotor nerves through the posterior longitudinal bundle.

THE PHYSIOLOGY OF OCULAR MOVEMENTS

Ocular movements in various directions are referred to be the ones initiating from the primary position.

1. *Primary position*: The eyes are looking straight ahead, the visual axes are parallel, the vertical meridians of corneas are vertical and parallel, and the head is vertical.
2. *Secondary position*: These are the positions of the eyes assumed when the eyes are moved around the transverse, vertical or anteroposterior axis.
3. *Tertiary position*: These positions are assumed when the eyes are moved along an oblique axis. Two laws govern the movements of the eyes into the tertiary position. These are:
   i. *Dander's law*: "For any determinate position of the line of fixation with respect to the head, there corresponds a definite and invariable angle of torsion, independent of the volition of the observer, and independent of the manner in which the line of fixation has been brought into the position in question". More simply stated, it is that for every rotation of the eye to a tertiary position there is a definite and measurable amount of torsion.
   ii. *Listing's law*: When the line of fixation passes from its primary to any other position, the angle of torsion of the eye in this second position is the same as if the eye had arrived at this position by turning about a fixed axis perpendicular to the initial and final positions of the line of fixation. In other words, in rotation to a tertiary position the eye will turn about that oblique axis which is perpendicular to the initial and final positions of the line of fixation.

Ocular Movements

The ocular movements may be described as monocular (ductions) or binocular (versions and vergences). Ductions include the following movements:

1. *Adduction*: An inward movement of the eye towards the nose, a medial rotation along the vertical axis.
2. *Abduction*: An outward movement, a lateral rotation along the vertical axis.

3. *Supraduction (Sursumduction)*: An upward movement or elevation along the horizontal axis.
4. *Infraduction*: When the eye moves down (depression) along the horizontal axis.
5. *Incycloduction (intorsion)*: When the eye makes a rotatory movement along the anteroposterior axis such that the superior pole (12 O'clock point) rotates towards the nose.
6. *Excycloduction (extorsion)*: When the eye rotates in a manner that the 12 O'clock point rotates away from the nose.

Versions (Conjugate movements)

These are synchronous and symmetric movements of both eyes in the same direction. These are classified according to the direction of binocular movements as follows **(Fig. 3.1).**

1. *Dextroversion*: When both eyes are turned to the right. It is affected by a simultaneous contraction of right lateral and left medial rectus muscle.
2. *Levoversion*: When both eyes are turned towards left by contraction of left lateral and right medial rectus.
3. *Supraversion*: When both eyes are rotated straight up. It is affected by a simultaneous contraction superior rectus and inferior oblique of both eyes.
4. *Infraversion*: When both eyes are turned straight down, and is caused by a bilateral contraction of inferior rectus and superior oblique muscles.

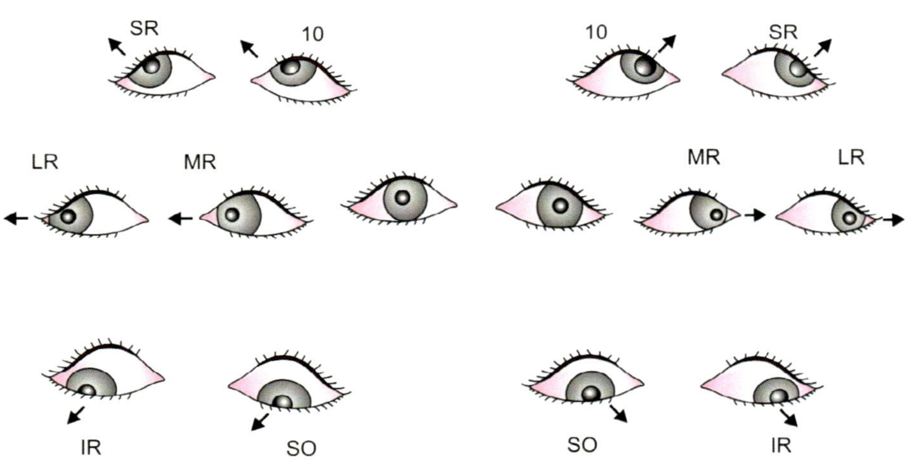

FIG. 3.1: Conjugate ocular movements

5. *Dextrodepression*: When both eyes are turned down and to the right. It is caused by a simultaneous contraction of right inferior rectus and left superior oblique.
6. *Dextroelevation*: When both eyes are turned up and to the right. It is caused by a simultaneous contraction of right superior rectus and left inferior oblique.
7. *Levoelevation*: When both eyes are turned up and to the left, a position achieved by a simultaneous contraction of left superior rectus and right inferior oblique.
8. *Levodepression*: When both eyes are turned down and to the left. This position is brought about by a simultaneous contraction of left inferior rectus and right superior oblique.
9. *Dextrocyclovesion*: When the eyes rotate along the anteroposterior axis so that the superior pole (12 O'clock point) rotates to the right side. This movement is brought about a simultaneous contraction of inferior rectus and inferior oblique muscle of the right eye, and superior rectus and the superior oblique of left eye.
10. *Levocycloversion*: A movement just opposite of dextrocycloversion.

Vergences

Vergences are disjugate, synchronous and symmetric movements of both eyes in the opposite direction. Depending upon the direction of movement vergences may be described as follows:

1. *Convergence*: It is a synchronous inward movement of both eyes brought about by a simultaneous contraction of both medial recti.
2. *Divergence*: It is a simultaneous and synchronous outward movement of both eyes brought about by a simultaneous contraction of both lateral recti. All ocular movements take place around a hypothetical point-center of rotation which lies 13.5 mm behind the apex of cornea. Though located slightly posterior, for practical purposes, it may be considered to coincide with the geometrical center of the eyeball. All rotations of the eyeball take place along three axes—Tick's axes which are perpendicular to each other and intersect at the center of rotation. These axes are:
   - X *Horizontal axis*: It lies horizontally when the head is in upright position. Rotation along this axis results in elevation or depression.
   - Y *Anteroposterior axis*: It lies anteroposteriorly and at right angle to the horizontal axis. The axes in the two eyes are parallel. Rotation along this axis results in torsional movements (extorsion and intorsion).

Z *Vertical axis*: It lies vertically when the head is in upright position, and is at right angle to the X and Y axis. Rotation along this axis causes adduction or abduction.

The ocular movements may be of two types — voluntary and involuntary. The latter are either fusional or due to vestibule ocular reflexes.

Voluntary

1. *Dextroversion and levoversion*: When both eyes are turned to the right or left respectively.
2. *Supraversion and infraversion*: When both eyes are turned up or down respectively.
3. *Oblique parallel movements*: When both eyes are turned up and right (Dextroelevation), up and left (levoelevation), down and right (Dextrodepression), down and left (levodepression).
4. *Convergence*: When both eyes are turned in during the process of converging on the point of fixation. This is essentially an involuntary phenomenon, but can also be achieved by a conscious effort.

Involuntary

1. Psychoptic reflexes, such as fixation, fusional movements, convergence, etc.
2. Statokinetic reflexes coordinate the position of the eyes when the head is rotated in space.
3. Static reflexes coordinate the movements of the eyes in respect of the position of the head upon the body.

ACTIONS OF EXTRAOCULAR MUSCLES

The action of any muscle in moving the eye around the center of rotation, may be considered as a tangential force acting at the point at which the muscle first touches the sclera (the tangential point). Beyond this point, this changes constantly as the eyeball rotates, the remainder of the muscle is in actual contact with the globe. This position is the arc of contact **(Fig. 3.2)**. While the action of horizontal muscles is straightforward that is, turning the eyeball inwards (medial rectus) or outwards (lateral rectus), action of other recti and oblique muscles depends upon the line of fixation of the eye at the given moment. In primary position the action of various muscles is described in **Table 3.1.**

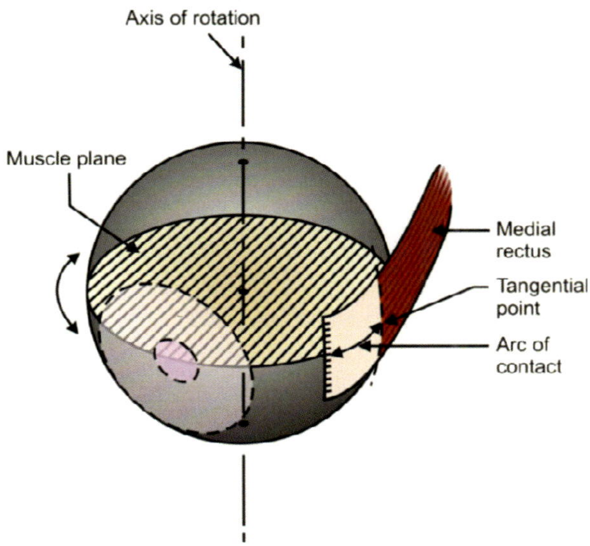

FIG. 3.2: Arc of contact

TABLE 3.1: Action of various muscles in primary position

Medial rectus	Adduction
Lateral rectus	Abduction **(Figs 3.3 to 3.5)**
Superior rectus	Elevation (Main action) Adduction and Intorsion (Subsidiary actions)
Inferior rectus	Depression (Main action) Adduction and Extorsion (Subsidiary actions)
Superior oblique	Intorsion (Main action) Depression and Abduction (Subsidiary actions)
Inferior oblique	Extorsion (Main action) Elevation and Abduction (Subsidiary actions)

To understand the mechanics of the main and subsidiary actions of the two vertical recti and the oblique muscles, it may be recalled that the vertical recti run forwards and laterally from their origin to the point of insertion, so that their anteroposterior axis lies at an angle of 23° with the visual axis. Secondly, the insertion of both muscles is anterior to the center of rotation. On contraction, the force of pull is directed from insertion towards the origin of the muscle. For example, the eye being in the primary position, contraction of superior rectus would cause a pull on the anterior pole upwards (elevation), as well as medially (adduction), and an internal rotation (intorsion). Similarly, a contraction

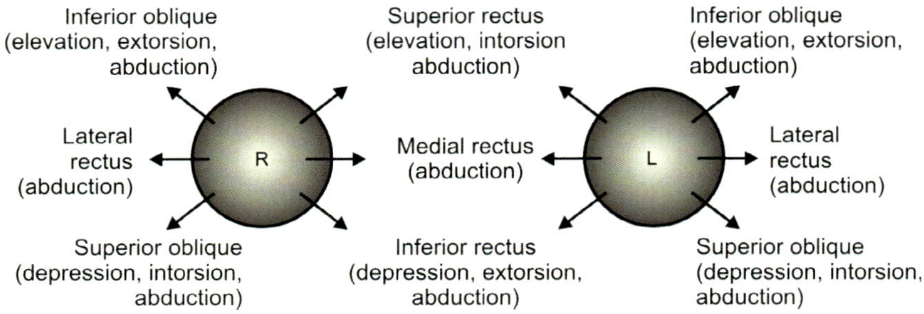

FIG. 3.3: Movement by each extrinsic ocular muscle

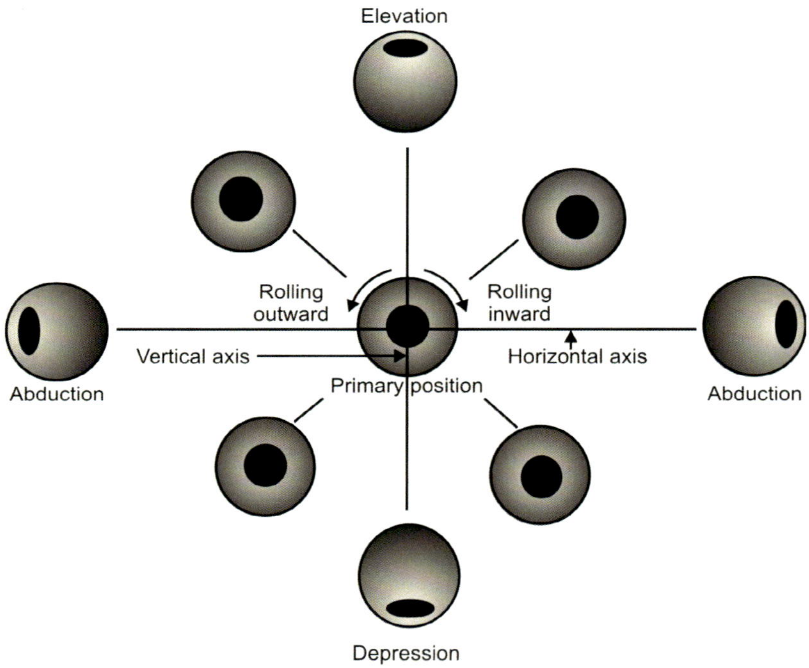

FIG. 3.4: Rotatory movement of eye

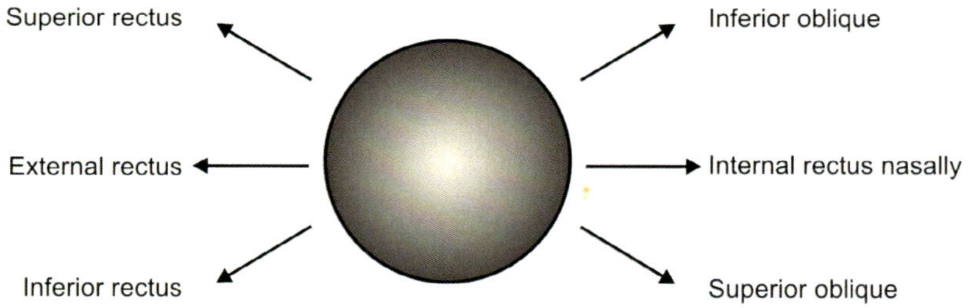

FIG. 3.5: Ocular movement

of inferior rectus muscle will affect a depression and adduction. But, being inserted on the inferior aspect of the globe it will cause rotation of the inferior pole inwards (thus causing an outward rotation of the superior pole-extorsion).

On the other hand if the eyeball is turned 23° outwards, the axes of the two recti shall coincide with the visual axis and the muscular contraction would cause maximal elevation or depression with a minimal amount of any subsidiary movement of adduction and torsion. If the globe could be turned in, at an angle of 67°, the plane of action of the two muscles would be perpendicular to the anteroposterior axis, the action of the muscles will be entirely torsion).

The actions of oblique muscles can be explained on a similar basis. Contrary to the recti the general direction of the oblique is from front backwards, the effective origin of the superior oblique being from the fibrous pulley at the upper and inner angle of the orbit. Secondly, both muscles are inserted behind the equator in the outer part of sclera. Thus contraction of superior oblique will pull the posterior pole up, causing a downward movement of the anterior pole (depression). Similarly the posterior pole will be pulled medially causing a movement of the anterior pole laterally (abduction). Its insertion being in the outer part of sclera, the pull of the muscle will tend to pull the globe inwards along the anteroposterior axis (intorsion). Likewise, contraction of inferior oblique will pull the posterior pole down (towards its origin) and hence the anterior pole up (elevation). The contraction will also pull the posterior pole medially and hence the anterior pole laterally (abduction). A rotation of the outer sclera (site of insertion) along the anteroposterior axis, shall be towards the floor of the orbit (extorsion).

The action of muscles described above are in the situation when the eyeball is in primary position. However if the globe is turned inwards making an angle of 51° with the visual axis, the plane of the obliques will coincide with the anteroposterior axis and the muscle will act purely as elevator or depressor with negligible subsidiary actions.

Thus, as far as elevation and depression are concerned, the obliques act when the eyeball is adducted while superior and inferior recti act when the ball is abducted. In the primary position, the recti are responsible for 63.3% of vertical motion while the obliques are responsible for 36.7%. An understanding of these actions is important in functional testing of vertical plane muscles.

In accordance with the action of an individual muscle uniocularly or in relation to the action of other muscles in the same eye or the contralateral eye the muscles can be classified as follows:

1. *Agonist*: It refers to a particular muscle causing a specific ocular movement. For example, in rotation of the eyeball to the left, lateral rectus of the left eye is agonist.
2. *Synergists*: The set of muscles which move the same eye in one particular direction are called synergists. For example, superior rectus and inferior oblique of the same eye are synergists in the movement of elevation of that eye.
3. *Antagonists*: These are the muscles having opposite action in the same eye, such as medial and lateral rectus.
4. *Yoke muscles* (contralateral synergists): This constitutes a pair of muscles (one in each eye) which contract synchronously and simultaneously to achieve any position of version. For example, left lateral rectus and right medial rectus contract simultaneously to achieve levoversion. The pair of yoke muscles would be different cardinal positions of gaze, as described in **Table 3.2**.

TABLE 3.2: Yoke muscles for different versions

Cardinal direction of gaze	*Pair of yoke muscles*
Dextroversion	Right Lateral Rectus Left Medial Rectus
Levoversion	Left Lateral Rectus Right Medial Rectus
Dextroelevation	Right Superior Rectus Left Inferior Oblique
Levoelevation	Left Superior Rectus Right Inferior Oblique
Dextrodepression	Right Inferior Rectus Left Superior Oblique
Levodepression	Left Inferior Rectus Right Superior Oblique

The pattern of innervation to various synergists and antagonist muscles is governed by two laws:

1. *Hering's Law of Equal Innervation*: According to this law an equal and simultaneous innervation flows from the brain to a pair of yoke muscles which contract simultaneously in different binocular movements. For example, in rotating the eyes to the position of dextroversion an equal and simultaneous energy will flow to right

lateral rectus and left medial rectus. Similarly, if the eyes are turned the position of dextroelevation an equal and simultaneous amount of energy (innervation) will flow to right superior rectus and left inferior oblique.

2. *Sherrington's Law of Reciprocal Innervation*: This law states that during an ocular movement an increased amount of innervation flow to the agonist muscle is accompanied by a decreased amount of innervation to the relaxing antagonist muscle. Thus, on moving the eyes to the right (dextroversion) an increased amount of innervation to the right lateral rectus and left medial rectus will be accompanied by a decreased amount of innervation to the right medial rectus and left lateral rectus.

The resultant clinical picture following an extraocular muscle palsy is influenced by this set of laws and will be discussed subsequently under the head—Paralytic Squint.

4 Binocular Vision

The two eyes being located some distance away from each other, image of any object formed in each eye cannot be identical, as each eye regards a slightly different aspect of the object observed. But the two slightly dissimilar images are mentally fused into a single image. In addition, such a fusion provides the perception of a third dimension to the image-stereopsis one of the greatest advantages of binocular vision. There are many factors involved in the successful development of binocular vision, which consist of complex and closely related sensory, motor and central mechanisms.

MECHANISMS

Sensory Mechanisms

Retinal Sensitivity

The two eyes should have a reasonably good and equal visual acuity. The refractive status of the two eyes may not be very different so that the images formed do not differ greatly.

Retinal Correspondence

Normally, any point of retinal receptors in one eye corresponds to another point in the other eye. For example, a point located 10° on the nasal side of one retina corresponds to another point located 10° placed temporarily in the other. Foveas in the two eyes provide the best example of corresponding points. Such points do not refer to individual retinal receptors but a group of receptors in a small area—Pannum area. Each eye contains many such areas and the sum of points in space the images will fall upon corresponding retinal areas is called horopter. In other words horopter can be considered as a sum total of points in the physical space that stimulate corresponding elements of two eyes. Conversely, an object which does not lie on the horopter forms image on noncorresponding points of the retina of two eyes, and if attention is directed to this object it would look double-Diplopia, which may be homonymous or crossed.

Visual Pathways

The development of binocular vision is dependent on a hemidecussation of the afferent optic nerve fibers at the optic chiasma because this enables the nerve fibers from corresponding retinal areas of the two eyes to become associated with one and other in the visual cortex. The retina may be divided, from the functional point of view, to be divided vertically through the midpoint of fovea. All retinal fibers from the temporal half of the retina including the temporal half of fovea pass through the chiasma without decussation, traveling along the ipsilateral optic tract. On the other hand, all retinal fibers from the nasal of the retina including the nasal half of fovea decussate at the chiasma and travel along the contralateral optic tract. It follows therefore, that fibers from the corresponding retinal areas (temporal retina of one eye and nasal retina of the other eye) travel in the same optic tract, terminate in the same lateral geniculate body, getting relayed to the same side of optic radiations to reach the striate area of the same visual cortex.

Motor Mechanisms

These are responsible for maintaining the eyes in the correct position at all times, i.e. inrest and during all movements, and may be considered in three groups:

Anatomical Factors

These are concerned with the structure of the bony orbits and their contents as well as the structure of the two eyeballs so that the eyes may lie within orbits in a manner that the visual axes be parallel to each other in all states of rest and various movements.

Physiological (or dynamic) Factors

These are the postural reflexes (static, statokinetic) which determine the position of eyes and are independent of visual stimuli. In addition, certain psychoptic reflexes make a significant contribution to the achievement of binocular vision, such as:

i. *Fixation reflex*: This relates to the ability of each eye to independently fix at the same object. It is dependent mainly on adequately functioning fovea and to some extent, on an adequate field of vision.

ii. *Refixation reflex*: This is an elaboration of fixation reflex, and consists of the ability of the two eyes to change fixation from one object to the other object (active refixation), or the ability of eyes to retain fixation of a moving object (passive refixation).

iii. *Disjunctive or vergence fixation reflex*: This the application of fixation reflex in which the eyes retain fixation during the course of a disjunctive movement such as convergence or divergence.

Central Mechanisms

These concern the development of fusion, which, though partly a sensory phenomenon, also partly concerns the cortical control of ocular movements which is a motor function. Perception of a single mental impression of two slightly different images as seen by the two eyes, is an essential part of the functions of visual cortex. The motor component of the phenomenon concerns the centers in the frontal and occipital parts of the central hemispheres which control the intermediary centers and the cranial nuclei concerned in the final impulses controlling the movements of extraocular muscles.

GRADES OF BINOCULAR VISION

The phenomenon of binocular vision has three different components:

Simultaneous Perception

This is the first grade of binocular vision. It refers to the simultaneous perception of the impulses, received from the two eyes, by the cerebral cortex. It is the faculty to see two dissimilar objects simultaneously. It does not necessarily mean that the image of two different objects concerned can be superimposed. This grade of binocular vision can be demonstrated on a major amblyoscope by using slides of two different pictures like a lion and a cage presented to the eyes individually. Simultaneous binocular perception can be:

i. Simultaneous paramacular perception

ii. Simultaneous macular perception

iii. Simultaneous foveal perception.

Under certain conditions human being have the faculty to suppress the image of one eye, though both eyes are open, such as looking through a monocular microscope, or shooting with a gun.

Fusion

This second grade of binocular vision. This is the faculty of producing a composite picture of two similar objects, each of which is incomplete in a different manner. When picture of two rabbits (one with a bunch of flowers in hand but without the tail, and the other with the tail but without flowers) is seen on a major amblyoscope, a single picture of the rabbit is seen in a complete form with a tail as well as a bunch of flowers in hand.

Fusion can be of two types:

i. Central
ii. Peripheral fusion.

Stereopsis

It is the highest form of binocular cooperation that adds a new quality of vision. It refers to the ability to obtain an impression of depth by the superimposition of two pictures of the same object taken from a slightly different angle. It is not just the depth perception which concerns the perceptions of distance between the objects, which can be judged even on a monocular vision. But stereopsis refers to the visual appreciation of three dimensions during binocular vision. Various tests to judge the quality of this faculty are described in subsequent chapters.

5 Visual Acuity

Visual acuity is defined as the power to differentiate object from each other and to appreciate their details. It is highly complex function consisting of:

i. The ability to detect an object in the field of vision.
ii. The ability to name a symbol or specify the position of a critical element in it.

Optically, the visual acuity is expressed as the minimum visual angle substended at the anterior focal plane when accommodation is entirely relaxed. Binocular visual acuity is always better than the monocular acuity.

Basically, the visual process can be considered as the reception of information by the retina, and the transmission of that coded information along the optic nerves and radiations to the cerebral cortex. The eye sees nothing as it is simply the input mechanisms of computer. Perception is the read-out mechanisms of that computer. It is of course the cortex alone which sees. Vision is a continuous process of receiving, sampling, analysing and coding information until the final decoding and read-out mechanism occurs. The pupillary reflex is present at birth demonstrating that neonate is sensitive to differences in intensity of the visual stimuli cortical cells in immature kitten leave a normal receptive field arrangement before their eyes are opened, demonstrating that patterned light stimuli are not necessary for the development of the functional architecture of the cerebral cortex.

Infants as young as 15 days can discriminate colors. By 1 month of age an infant sees complex forms and can see the difference between a gray patch and square composed of 3mn stripes. By the age of 6 months a baby's coordination has reached a stage where he will repeat responses which produce interesting results, such as swinging a toy, and clearly to do this, his vision must have developed accordingly. So that fixation and following movement occur as well as the recognition of familiar and interesting objects. By a month baby will knock down pillow to find a toy and he is able visually to differentiate objects easily. As age increases, through trial and error experiment (11-18 months) and later thinking about the effects of various responses (18-24 months) the child builds up his memory store so that at 12-18 months he will look for an object hidden under a second pillow and at 18-24 months he will look for the object even when it has been removed.

Thus, with increasing age the percepts breaks up and instead of seeing things as a whole, he is able to differentiates the stimuli in his surroundings, the percept can begin to be seen as its components parts. Discrimination of symbol and letters develops gradually so that by the age of 1 years a child can distinguish simple symbols and by 5 or 6 years he can distinguish letters.

At birth foveal sensitivity and the cortical control behind it is not well-developed. It is by continued use and by the reception of repeated and useful information, that the cortex is able to program itself and build up a satisfactory memory alone, so that it is able to compare data samples presented to it and increase its ability. At first a lot of data, is required to produce a simple response.

The infant will respond simply to complex colored, patterns and shapes. As age increase, and with, repeated stimulation the cortical cells increase the selectivity of their response in infancy. Visual sensitivity is recognized by means of pupillary reflexes demonstrating integrity of the nervous pathway to the lateral geniculate body, and later, by the response to complex forms, demonstrating integrity of the prewired mechanism of the cortex.

This is followed by recognition of complex forms, demonstrating integrity of an elementary memory store for perception. Presentation of symbols containing the same amount of information within decreasing areas gives us our test of visual acuity. By the time a child is 3 years he can distinguish and demonstrate his acuity by recognition of such symbols.

It should be realized that 6/9 using a simple symbol does not necessarily mean that the vision will be 6/9 after further development of the visual mechanism using more complex tests. If the vision is 6/9 at 3 years of age using symbols than one expects it to be 6/9 with Snellen's test at 6 year. But this assumes a normal development of the cortex and retina. The excellence of Snellen's test of vision is due to these factors, large amount of information is packed into a confined area and the area containing this information can be varied easily. It is not until a child can read line of 6/6 Snellen letter at a resonable speed that we can be certain that the visual mechanism is normal. 6/6 visions determines the ability of the sensitivity curve of the fovea. The speed at which the line can be read determines the effectiveness of the position control system of that sensitivity curve and the ability of whole decoding mechanism of the visual cortex.

ANGULAR AND CORTICAL VISUAL ACUITY

The response to a single optotype has been termed angular vision, while the response to a row of letter is known as cortical vision, the reading of a row of letter involves interpretation by the cortex, whereas angular vision, or recognizing simple optotypes, depends simply on the angular magnification of the letter. It is obvious that all visual processes must involve cortical activity, the eye is only the axons by which visual sensations are transmitted to the cortex. We do not see through one eye or through both eyes, but through the brain as through Cyclopean eye.

RECORDING OF VISUAL ACUITY

Snellen visual acuity represents the patient's resolving capability on letter targets. Vernier visual acuity is a test of resolving minimal separations of a grid pattern. The essence of both these methods of testing visual acuity is that an object subtends different angles on the retina when presented at different distances from the eye.

The angle subtended by the object at the nodal point of the eye is called the visual angle. Visual resolution is measured by the angle at which the components of an object can be appreciated. They are commonly measured in minutes of arc and decimal fractions of minutes. The Snellen notation 6/6 means that the subject can read letters composed of black lines on a white background 6 meter away when the width of each line subtends 1 minutes of arc on the retina.

The notation 6/12 correspondents to 2 minutes of arc the Snellen notation, therefore, can be expressed by the formula.

$$\text{Visual angle (minutes)} = 1 \ / \ \text{Snellen notation}$$

Occasionally, the Snellen notation is expressed as a decimal fraction, thus 6/6 is 1.0, 6/12 is 0.5 and so on. The smallest detectable visual angle has been found to be 0.5 second of arc against a uniformly illuminated background such a line producer a geometric retinal image approximately 0.033 mm, which is the diameter of single foveal cone. "Snellen's chart" should be accepted as international chart to determine the subjective visual acuity. Each component of top letter of Snellen's chart subtends an angle of vision at 60 meters. Whole the letter in the line indicating normal visual acuity (6/6) subtend the same angle at a distance of 6 meters. Six meters is accepted from practical point of view because most rays from a distance of 6 meter and more are as good as parallel rays. Depending on the number of lines the patient can read, distance vision is recorded as 6/60 to 6/6 with Snellen's chart illuminated either externally or internally with uniform illumination. The intensity of the light over the chart should be between 20 to 30 foot candles in a diffuse manner and at the same time there should be no brilliant light in the visual field of the patient. The chart is placed over a white wall, or if it is necessary, it can be mounted on top of white paper. The chart is placed in such a manner that the eyes of the patients one level with the 20/20 line. The patients can be standing or sitting. The chart can be elevated or lowered according to the different heights of the patients. A line is made at 20 feet from the chart, and if the person to be tested is standing his head should be at the level of the line. Some chart even have letter for recording visual acuity up to 6/5 to 6/4. If a person misses, or incorrectly reads some letters of a line, the record is qualified as 'partial'. Farther more vision should be recorded for each eye separately as well as binocularly. It is to be noted that the binocular vision (both eyes open) is always one line more than the uniocular vision provided both eyes have equal visual acuity.

The macular part of the retina is most sensitive part and most visual acuity is derived from this area. Retinal sensitivity gradually diminishes from the center to the periphery, so much so that the peripheral retina has only 10% of the central sensation. It is an every day experience that a person with a gross localized foveal lesions with whole of the remaining retina normal will not have visual acuity more than 6/60 or 6/36 partial. On the other hand with gross pathological lesions in peripheral retina but an unaffected macular area, patient may have 6/6 vision, although this will be tubular in character because of the loss of peripheral field. In the grades of vision take 6/60, 6/36.............6/9, 6/6 the constant number 6 in the numerator indicates the distance from which patient is reading and the denominator indicates the distance in meters from which the patient should be able to read that line. Countries not following the metric system denote it is feet as 20/200 to 20/20.

If the vision with both eyes open is 3/60 or less (with correction if necessary), it is total blindness because a person with that poor visual acuity cannot independently move about except in very familiar surroundings. If vision, again with both eyes open, and with correction, if necessary, is more that 3/60 but 6/60 or less, it is considered economic blindness, because such a person by virtue of his visual cannot earn his living independently, vision better that 6/60 but 6/18 or less again with both eyes open and with correction is considered a visual handicap because such a person is visually handicapped and may be unfit for service or jobs needing good visual acuity.

Three types of charts are being used for illiterate pupil. The Landolt's 'C' charts are accepted as standard for testing visual acuity for various progressive in preference to others. The 'E' charts are also identical and can be used under the same guidelines as 'C' charts. The dot charts showing different number of dots of different sizes are also covenant. Multicolored balls can be used from different distances for the toddlers.

It is rarely possible to obtain any significant subjective responses for visual acuity determination of children under the age of 3 years and hence recourse has to be made entirely to the objective methods assessment. Quantitative upto kinetic test can be carried out with most small children. Visual four test pattern equal width of 1/8,1/16. 1/32 and 1/64 inches mounted on the C, K, N drum. At the test distance of 12 inches they represent 36, 18,9 and 4.5 minutes of visual angle. The level of illumination was set at 100 foot candles. Minimum separable acuity threshold were established by observing prompt and properly directed rhythmic optokinetic responses in both direction of the rotation of the cylinder in eight out of ten trials with each test pattern.

Forced choice preferential looking test by employing patterns and acuity grating is useful in infants and young children. This test allows the child to look at screens while observing the behavior of the eye and head.

Normal adult acuity can be attained by 4-5 months. This can be elicited by visual evoked responses (VEH) to square move gratings of various spatial frequencies.

VISION IN VARIOUS REFRACTIVE ERRORS

Hypermetropia

The uncorrected visual acuity in hypermetropes varies with the degree of optical error and the portion which cannot be overcome by accommodation.

The corrected visual acuity frequently does not come upto standard, particularly in higher degrees of the defect, usually when the refractive error was not corrected in early childhood (Ametropic amblyopia) but the acuity improves to same extent after wearing correcting spectacles for some months. Hypermetropes who do not wear correcting spectacles or wear them intemittently. See better without them. A variable incidence of amblyopia has been reported. The commonest cause of such a condition is hypermetropic refractive error and amblyopia could be prevented by early use of glasses.

Myopia

Visual acuity beyond the far point is seriously affected in incorrected myopia, being reduced by about the same ratio as in hypermetropia. The corrected visual acuity in the absence of degenerative changes is usually good and even better with contact lenses. Individual who use spectacles habitually see less well without them than those who do wear them intermittently or not at all incidence of amblyopia in myopia is much less almost unknown for the reason that myopia at least sees the near objects more clearly than in hypermetropia where all accommodation reserve is up for distance and he neither sees distance nor see near objects clearly. Therefore, near vision stimulus is not derived in myopia.

Astigmatism

The vision in astigmatism is characteristic. In higher degree of astigmatism eye cannot form a sharply defined image on the retina in any circumstance, therefore, vision may be diminished very considerably. The dimension of visual acuity is about equal for corresponding degree of simple hypermetrope and myopia astigmatism can usually be brought upto normal standard. But in higher degrees this is by no means always the case particularly if the optical correction is not made early life and also if the astigmatism is oblique. This deficiency is essentially perceptual and there may be a tendency for poor differentiation in the meridian of greatest astigmatism. Astigmatic amblyopia or meridional amblyopia is present then. Amblyopia ex-anopsia affecting all meridia is more common in higher degrees of astigmatism and there is a tendency to develop strabismus particularly in the presence of hypermetropic errors.

Anisometropia

Binocular vision is the rule in smaller degree of the defect with higher grades of error, fusion is usually impossible and alternating and unocular vision may occur. Alternating vision may result in which case each of the two eyes is used one at a time and is specially so if both eyes have good visual acuity and when one is hemitropic or moderately hypermetropic and other is myopic. The patient uses the former for distant vision and latter for near vision. He may therefore remain very comfortable and at times be unaware of the defect. If the defect in one eye is high and especially if the visual acuity is not good it may be altogether excluded from vision and the better eye is relied upon in unocular vision.

OBSTACLES TO VISION AT VARIOUS AGES FROM BIRTH TO INFANCY

The fixation reflex is innate being present at birth but is only feebly developed, responding momentarily to strong stimulus such as bright light, in general. The movements of the eyes are independent irregular and unconjugated. Obstacles to vision at birth lead to failure in development of fixation and congenital nystamus results. By the age of 5 or 6 weeks the conjugate fixation reflex becomes established but it is not until almost 6 months that conjugate deviations become completely accurate. Owing to the inter position of some obstacles in the reflex path, fusion may be embarrassed and maintained with difficulty, resulting in heterophoria later: squint or not attained at all resulting into concomitant squint. Again some structural obstacles (neuromuscular) may prohibit the development of adequate conjugate movements from birth, so that a congenital nondominant squint develops. Desjugate fixation reflexes are developed after 6 months. Failure of the desjugate fixation reflexes are firmly established towards the end of the first year and if obstacles become insuperable diplopia results.

If there would be obstacle to any of the reflexes developing at various ages, various types of neuromuscular anomalies would develop. Apart from, this, the visual acuity may be permanently impaired if there is any obstacle whether refractive error, strabismus, congenital cataract and ptosis. The amount and density of amblyopia would thus depend on the visual acuity that has developed by that age.

6 Abnormalities of Binocular Vision

The binocular reflexes may be greatly modified by the presence of obstacle in the reflex path. Although these obstacles are more hundering when reflexes are immature, they can even interference with the fully developed reflexes. The presence of these abnormal obstacles results in the development of perverted reflexes, any of structural anomalies, which replace the normal. The younger the patient, the more likely is a slight obstacle to produce a permanent effect.

There obstacle may be divided into sensory, motor and central. The penalty suffered by an adult through such a simple sensory obstacle as incorrect glasses may not exceed headache and various irritability, but a child in such a circumstances may have pay with his sight. A careful consideration of motor obstacles isolate large group of paralytic squint from what has ordinary concomitant squint. The chief factor in incomplicated accommodational squint is a congenital and hereditary deformity, excessive hypermetropia, and the factor next in importance is weakness of the neuromuscular mechanism of accommodation. The resulting insufficiency of accommodation axial on one hand and dynamic on other hand, instead of being overcome by the occipital accommodation reflex alone, elicits an attempt at correction by a frontal effort which ensues as accommodation and convergence in abnormal association, excessive convergence resulting in a, attempt to over-accommodation.

According to chavasse, in any case of dissociation whether this is due to a sensory or a motor obstacle, two vicious circles, linked together as a figure of eight, are in action, whether the type of deviation is concomitant, paralytic or mixes. Whatever the cause of dissociation changes rapidly develop as shown in **Figure 6.1.**

MECHANISM

According to von Noorden, whenever there is a manifest deviation of the visual axes of the two eyes, the images of all objects in the binocular

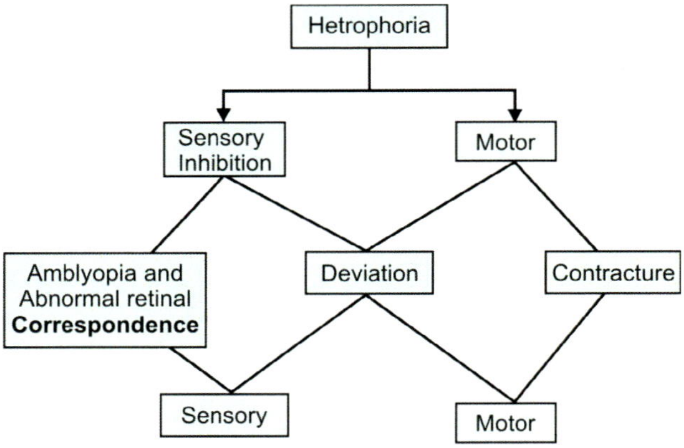

FIG. 6.1: Chavasse vicious circle

field are shifted on the two retinal relative to each other, the larger the shift, the grater the deviation. Motor and sensory fusion may become impossible with two distressing results. Different objects are imaged on corresponding areas (that is, the two foveas) and therefore are seen in the same visual direction and overlap identical objects (that is the fixation points) are imaged on disparate retinal areas (that is fovea of one eye and the peripheral retina of the other eye) and, therefore are seen in different visual directions and appear double. The first phenomenon is turned confusion and the second, diplopia.

Any factor which hampers the development of binocular reflexes before they get fully established can lead to development of concomitant squint.

Binocular Vision and Anisometropia

Binocular vision is a complex phenomenon, which is possible in human beings only due to development of some anatomical and physiological factors. It provides wider field of vision, excludes the overlapping of monocular defects and above all provides a stereopic vision.

Good visual acuity, normal physiological retinal correspondence, proper coordination and fixation with each eye, formed, are the essential requirements of binocular vision. This being an acquired phenomenon any obstacle during its development may hinder binocular vision, Anisometropia is one of the most important dioptric obstacle in this regard. Anisometropia affects binocular vision in the following ways.

1. Formation of blurred image in more ametropic eye and a sharp image in the emmetropic eye causes a sensory obstacle for fusion.

2. Unequal size of the retinal images (Aniseikonia) causes difficulty in fusion.
3. Prismatic effect due to unequal power of the correcting spectacles causes unequal peripheral fusion.
4. Difficulty in binocular—spatial judgment because of aniseikonia.

A blurred image and aniseikonia may lead to the development of foveal suppression, amblyopia, abnormal retinal correspondence and strabismus. It has been observed that if a patient of anisometropia is having binocular vision and if given treatment for amblyopia he improves by better visual status and longer maintenance than those cases who lack binocular function. In few cases, if aniseikonia and prismatic effect are overcome by using contact lenses, there patients maintain good binocular vision.

There is no rigid relationship between anisometropia and aniseikonia. It has generally accepted that 25 diopter difference of refraction causes 0.5% differences in image size.

Vision in Anisometropia

The vision in significant anisometropia may be binocular, alternating or exclusively uniocular.

a. *Binocular vision:* Binocular vision is noticed in smaller degree of anisometropia.

   Each 0.25D difference between the refraction of the two eyes causes 0.5> difference in the size between the two retinal images. Probably the difference of 5D is the limit which can usually be tolerated with case. Moreover since the incorrected image of one eye is always blurred binocular vision is rarely perfect, and attempts of fusion frequently, although not always, bring on symptoms of accommodative asthenopia. The symptomatology of this group thus resembles that of small refractive errors.

b. *Alternating vision:* This occur in higher degrees of anisometropia, here each of the two eyes is used one at a time. This is apt to occur when the visual acuity of both the eyes are good and one is emmetropic or moderately hypermetropic and other myopic. Here the patient falls into the easy and legitimate habit of using the eye which is emmetropic or hypermetropic for the distant vision and the other eye which is myopic for near work, and he may remain very comfortable and indeed quiet unaware of his defect and if the anisometropia is mixed, require no optical correction for any distance at any time of life.

c. *Uniocular vision (Suppression):* If the refractive error in one is very high and if its visual acuity is poor, it may be altogether excluded from the vision and the other eye alone being relied upon in uniocular vision. In this event the defective eye may become not a uncommonly deviated.

Relationship between Anisometropia and Amblyopia

Visual acuity in the anisometropic eye is lower under binocular conditions then when tested monocularly. This is because of the fact that in anisometropic patients, the purpose of active inhibition of fovea is to eliminate sensory interference caused by super imposition of a focused and a defocused image originating from the fixation point (abnormal binocular interaction). Apart from this the foveal form vision-deprivation due to uncorrected refractive error plays a role in producing amblyopia. After optical correction of anisometropia, the resulting aniseikonia may be another causal factor of amblyopia.

Intensity of amblyopia rended to very directly with the amount of anisometropia. Amblyopia is more common and a higher degree in patients with anisohypermetropia than in those with anisomyopia. Retina of the more ametropic of a pair of hypermetropia eyes never receives clearly defined image, since with details clearly focused on the fovea of the better eye no stimulus is provided for the further accommodative effort required to produce a clear image in the fovea of the more hypermetropic eye when myopia is unequal, the more myopic eye can be used for near work and the less myopic eye for distance. Therefore, unless the myopia is of high degree both retinal receive adequate stimule and amblyopia does not develop. Apart from this, myopia is rarely present in early childhood, Amblyopia frequently occurs when the degree of anisometropia is higher than 2.0.

In anisometrop amblyopia the central suppression scotoma is normally small so that the optic phenomenon of Haidinger's brushes may be obtain able, a capacity which indicates that the prognosis after treatment is relatively good.

Relationship with Squint

In anisometropia the influence which accommodation convergence relationship may exert on development of squint depends largely on whether one is used constantly for fixation irrespective of distance of gaze or whether one eye is used for fixation for near objects and the other eye for fixation for those situated at a distance. When one eye is dominant and has only a moderate degree of hypermetropia the other eye tends to remain straight irrespective of wheather it is more hypermetropic or less hypermetropic than the dominant eye or even when it is myopic, a clear illustration of the fact that in early infancy the eyes are associated with one another by the more primitive postural reflexes without any regard to the presence of a high refractive error in one eye. When one eye is dominant and has a fairely marked degree of hypermetropia, the other eye may remain straight or may tend to diverge when either eye is dominant so that one eye is used for distance and the other eye for near, divergence may occur because there is not reward to be obtained from the exercise of accommodation convergence reflex. Anisometropia also constitutes a central obstacle of a sensory type. There is also evidence that errors of refraction even fully corrected by spectacle lenses, may favor the development of squint in certain cases when there is moderate degree of difference between the refraction of the two eyes (anisometropia) leading to a sufficient size difference of the retinal images (aniseikonia) which prevent the normal fulfilment of fusion mechanism despite the clarity of each separate image in the visual cortex. In such cases a positive attempt to prevent fusion (a state termed horror fusion) may lead to the development of purposive strabismus.

It seems, likely therefore that a primary failure in the development of the fusion faculty plays significant part in the production of certain squint although it must be realized that in most of the cases the defect of fusion faculty is largely secondary to some motor or sensory obstacle so that the duration of the visual axes in the direct cause of the lack of reinforcement of the fusion reflex.

In unilateral myopia of moderate degree the myopia eye can diverge. In anisometropia of moderate degree in which one eye is myopic and other hypermetropic or relatively so, the myopic eye is usually used for near fixation and the hypermetropic eye for distance fixation in which case an alternating divergent strabismus develop.

Anisometropia and Eccentric Fixation

There are several hypothesis regarding the cause of eccentric fixation. According to "Scotoma hypothesis", central inhibitional scotoma or loss of macular function is the cause of eccentric fixation which develops similar to anomalous correspondence on the basis of constant deviation of the visual axis. Eccentric fixation and anomalous retinal correspondence (ARC) are only different stages of same pathophysiologic event occurring as an adoptation to faulty "binocular position". According to "motor-hypothesis", fixation is significantly influenced by motor factors.

7 Accommodative Convergence/ Accommodation Ratio

Whenever a person exerts a certain amount of accommodation a determined amount of convergence is called into play, called accommodative convergence. The convergence response of an individual to a unit stimulus of accommodation may be expressed in a number termed his accommodative convergence accommodation ratio. It is reasonable to assume that the basic convergence requirement is fulfilled through accommodative convergence. Tonic and fusional convergence have their own functions and proximal convergence is a supplementary one. Therefore a normal emmetropic person should be expected to exect IMA of convergence for each diopter of accommodation, but this is not the case. Each individual responds to a unit stimulus of accommodation with a specific amount of convergence that may be greater or smaller than is called for by the convergence requirement. The convergence response of an individual to a unit stimulus of accommodation may be expressed in a number termed accommodative convergence/accommodation ratio (AC/A ratio). This ratio which has the dimensions (D/D) is a measure of the responsiveness of person's convergence function to a unit of stimulation of accommodation. Quantitative studies on persons with normal sensorimotor system have shown that in the vast majority of people, the AC/A ratio does not fulfil the convergence requirement. The normal range of the AC/A ratio is between three and five. Values above five are considered to denote excessive accommodative convergence and values under three as in sufficiency.

The association between accommodation and convergence develops early in life as a result of constantly repeated simultaneous use of related degrees of the two functions, that is a learned association has been accepted and elaborated on by many workers. An acquired association implies a certain degree of independence in the relationship of two functions. This elastic relationship is expressed as "relative accommodation" and "relative convergence". Any change in the stimulus to accommodation that can be shown to lead to a change in convergence or that accommodation can be changed by forced convergence would favor an innate and stable relationship between the two types of convergence. Furthermore if the association is learned, one would not expect it to exist in patients who have had strabismus throughout most or all their lives. There is an increase in AC/A ratio in early presbyopia which is attributed to an increase in impulse to accommodation, somewhat similar to that required with cycloplegia. It is observed that AC/A is a factor in the inheritance of esotopia.

METHODS FOR DETERMINATION OF RATIO

Various methods are devised for measuring AC/A ratio

a. Heterophoric method
b. Gradient method
c. Fixation-desparity method
d. Haloscopic method
e. Graphic method.

Changes in AC/A ratio with glasses, drugs operation and exercise, both accommodation and convergence have a central and peripheral mechanism. There is a gradual decrease of esotropia. At near fixation without changes of the angle at distance in children wearing bifocal. It wears that spectacle lenses have changed AC/A ratio. It is demonstrated that AC/A ratio is reduced by using parasympathomimetic drug such as echothiophate iodide. This drug is cholinesterase inhibitor and it enhances the effect of acetylcholine on the ciliary muscle. There is a reduction in AC/A ratio by gradient method when the eyes were under the influence of di-iso-propyl fluorophosphates (DFP) and phospholine iodide (PI). This is because parasympathomimetic drugs affect the pupil. The greater depth of focus of an eye with a narrow pupil would reduce the need to accommodate and hence, reduce the accommodation effort. Weakening the action of the medial rectus muscle effect the AC/A ratio. This can be explained by a change in the relationship between muscular constructions and the resulting rotation of the eyes. Operations on the medial recti muscle reduces the mechanical effectiveness and the change is long lasting. Ethanol not only increases tonic convergence but also reduces AC/A ratio.

Generally, orthoptic exercise do not change AC/A ratio but sometimes in patients with exophoris orthoptic exercises induce a small increase in AC/A ratio.

Details of the Methods for Determination of AC/A Ratio

Heterophoria method is a useful and simple technique for determining the AC/A ratio in clinical practice. It is used in the evaluation of squints, particularly in deciding the nature of appropriate surgical intervention, long before the recognition of AC/A ratio as such.

In esodeviation, when the measurements for distance and near are equal, the AC/A ratio is normal and when the measurement for distance is greater than for near, the ratio is low. While in exodeviation it is high and when greater for near than distance the AC/A ratio high in esodeviation and low in exodeviation. But it must conceded that some degrees of difference possibly as much as 10° is within normal limits. In such patients, AC/A ratio as determined with gradient method is actually normal or may be subnormal and reliance on the heterophoric method will miss the correct diagnosis. Heterophoric method is useful and relatively simple method of determining the AC/A ratio in clinical practice. This consists of comparing the measurements of the latent deviation of the eyes, using the prism and alternate cover method, at a point of distant fixation (6 meters) and at a point of near fixation (1/3 meters) with care to ensure steady accommodation at both distance of fixation by the use of a target which contains detail, like a Snellen's test type letter, and with the use of an appropriate spectacle correction when there is any significant refractive error. It is possible to give the AC/A ratio a pricise value by the heterophoric method when account is taken of the interpupillary distance. In this way the AC/A ratio is equal to the interpupillary distance in centimeters plus the difference between the latent deviation in prism diopters for distance (at 6 meters) and for near (at 1/3 meter) after dividing this difference by the distance of the near fixation in diopter (that is, the amount of accommodation which is exerted at 1/3 meter by an emmetrope) or after multiplying it by the distance of the near fixation in meters. By this method:

$$AC/A = IPD + \frac{D2\text{-}D1}{F1} \quad \text{or} \quad AC/A = IPD + (D2 - D1) \times F2$$

Where,

AC = Accommodative convergence in prism diopters (D)
A = Accommodation in diopters (D)
IPD = Interpupillary distance in centimeters (cms)
D1 = Latent deviation for distance (6M)
D2 = Latent deviation for near (1/3 M)

F1 = Distance of near fixation in diopters
F2 = Distance of near fixation in meters

Example:

If IPD = 6 cm
D1 = 4 Dexo
D2 = 10 Dexo
F1 = 3 D
AC1A = 6 = (–10 – (–4)

$$\frac{6 + (-10 + 4)}{3}$$

= 6 + (–2)
= 4

Or if IPD = 6 cm
D1 = 4 Dexo
D2 = 10 Dexo
F2 = 1/3 M
AC/A = 6 + (–10 (–4) × 1/3
= 6 + (–10 + 4) × 1/3
= 6 – (–2)
= 4

THE MAJOR ABLYOSCOPIC METHOD

The instrument is adjusted to the patients interpupillary distance in the usual manner, the correcting spectacles are worn. Targets are used which ensure foveal fixation. The subjective angle is determined and the readings taken from the prism diopter scale. Minus lenses usually-3DS are inserted in the lens holder of the instrument and the measurement is repeated. The AC/A ratio is calculated from the following equation:

$$AC/A = \frac{D2 - D1}{D}$$

Where D1 is the subjective angle measured with patient's own spectacles

D2 is the subjective angle measured with addition of – 3 ODS
D is the strength in diopters of concave spherical lens used
e.g. If D2 = 19 Deso
D1 = 7 Deso
D = -3 OD Sph.
AC/A = +19. O – (+7) = + 12 = 4

This method is comparable to the gradient method when using Snellen's test types. The advantage of using this method is that small deviations can be more accurately measured than may be possible by means of the prism and cover test.

Graphic Method

By this method we measure the ratio and determine its character by using the major amblyoscope along with the graph. The aim of the test is to determine whether the accommodative convergence response is slow or rapid. Each measurement so obtained must be compared with normal convergence which accompanies each diopter of accommodation in the maintenance of binocular single vision, so that there is a direct comparison between this and the patient's subjective angle as recorded on the prism-diopter scale.

Method of Fixation Disparity

It is apparent that the magnitude of the fixation disparity gives information about a heterophoria. Which is not strickly comparable to that revealed by most other methods because it had the advantage of not creating dissociation of the eyes. It is possible also to change the state of the heterophoria by altering the vergence of the eyes by the use of prisms and of the accommodation by the use of spherical lenses. In this way the value of the muscular imbalance may be related to the accommodative convergence relationship so that is provides on assessment of the AC/A ratio.

There are several advantages in exploring AC/A ratio by the method of fixation disparity as compared with the others. Both eyes receive the same stimuli for accommodation both are subjected to the same type of estimation and fusion of the two eyes is maintained during the period of the test so that there is no element of dissociation of the eyes. But this is complicated and time consuming procedure and not suitable for routine clinical determinations particularly in young children.

Holoscopic Method

When the subject reads a line of fine print to maintain his/her accuracy of focusing, the deviation of the eyes and the degree of accommodation are measured simultaneously at different lavels. It is found that the deviation increases as the eye accommodates and is usually measured by the phoria for distant vision and also at the near point with the appropriate spectacle correction in place, the result is calculated by dividing the change of phoria from the one for the near distance by the diopteric change occurring between the two distances. Modern major amblyoscope is widely used for calculating this ratio.

Gradient Method

In determining the AC/A ratio by this method the change in the stimulus to accommodation is produced by means of ophthalmic lenses. For a given fixation distance minus lenses placed before the eyes increase the requirement for accommodation and plus lenses relax accommodation. It is assured that – 1D lenses produce an equivalent of 1D of accommodation whereas + lenses relax accommodation by 1D and that the accommodative response to the lenses is linear within a certain range. In the gradient method the AC/A ratio is measured by an estimation of the difference between the deviations of the eyes for a given distance using a Maddox rod in front of one eye and correcting prisms in front of other eyes go that there is change in their accommodation and therefore in their convergence. Convex lenses by decreasing the amount of accommodation necessary for the given distance decreases the amount of convergence and concave lenses by increasing the amount of accommodation increase the amount of convergence. The importance in determining there deviation of the eyes is to ensure that the patient exerts the full amount of accommodation required for the particular fixation distance. This is achieved best by the use of an object which contain much fine detail in conjunction with the alternate prism and cover test, in preference to the use simply of a fixation light as in the usual Maddox rod test. Difference of the deviation are measured by subtracting the first deviation from the second deviation, due regard to sign, plus measurements when esodeviation and minus when an exodeviation. The final figure of the ratio is obtained by dividing the difference in the deviations by the power of the lenses used, to reduce it to a simple unit of accommodation for the care of comparison. As a general rule the values for the AC/A ratio by this method are slightly lower than those obtained by the heterophoric method because the fix distances which is adopted throughout the gradient method precludes some of the influence of the factor of proximal convergence. This method has the advantage of inducing convergence which is mainly due to the patient's subjective accommodative error.

8 *Heterophoria*

Heterophoria/latent deviation is a condition of imperfect balance of the extrinsic ocular muscles in which there is a tendency if the eyes to deviate from their norm a relative position. This tendency, however, is kept in checked by the desire for binocular vision and by the reserve neuromuscular power of the eye.

Since the position of rest is usually of a slight divergence, only a few people are really orthophoric, hence some degree of heterophoria is universal.

CLASSIFICATION OF HETEROPHORIA

1. Exophoria
2. Esophoria
3. Hyperphoria
4. Hypophoria
5. Cyclophoria
   i. Incyclophoria
   ii. Excyclophoria

Exophoria is again divided into
   i. Divergence excesses
      Exphoria is greater for distance
   ii. Convergence weakness
      Exophoria is greater for near
   iii. Mixedor tonic

Esophoria is further divided into
   i. Convergence excess type
   ii. Divergence insufficiency type
   iii. Mixed type

ETIOLOGY OF HETEROPHORIA

Heterophoria can be classified into the following types.

Exophoria

Persistent use of accommodation by the hypermetropic favors the development of esophoria. There are two groups of causes for constant exophorias: (1) static causes and (2) anomalies of sensorimotor system. Innervational factors for causation of exophoria. Congenital abnormalities of orbit, e.g. in extreme forms of hypertelorism, a wide interpupillary distance is produced leading to exophoria. Exophoria may also occur in exophthalmos in which there is some displacement of the eyeball outwards. They also laid the emphasis of certain occupations, e.g. watchmaker or microscopist which entail prolonged uniocular activity tend to produce exophoria in later life which is accompanied by ocular neglect or suppression.

In the production of exophoria, AC/A ratio plays an important role. A high ratio with exophoria is sometimes seen in myopes due to the relative weakness of the response of the ciliary muscles compared with that of the medial recti. It is also sometimes seen in presbyopes in whom accommodation diminishes. In contrast, in exophoria (convergence weakness type) the AC/A ratio is usually low but may be normal in which an uncorrected refractive error may be an important influence in producing the exodeviation.

Esophoria

Persistent use of accommodation by the hypermetrope in excess of his convergence in order to attain clear vision favors the development of esophoria. On the other hand, in congenital or infantile myopia there is increased convergence leading to esodeviation. Due to central over activity through convergence impulses, esophoria is typically seen in energetic or unrestrained, in the young, strong, asthenic or neurotic in contrast with exophoria.

Esophoria could be produce if the orbits are set close together with a narrow interpupillary distance. The displacement of the eyeball inwards in cases of enophthalmos can lead to esophoria. They also regarded physiological defects (e.g. lack of coordination of reflexes associated with convergence or divergence) as cause of heterophoria and thus explained the basis of esophoria as an underlying cause of excessive application to close work. The most common factor etiologically to produce esophoria is an increased convergence innervation associated with increased accommodation determined either by a hypermetropic refractive error or arising from optical cause associated with accommodative strain.

Hyperphoria

Hyperphoria is of three different types with three different reasons.

Static Hyperphoria

It is due to the anatomical factors which determine the position of rest.

Paretic Hyperphoria

It is due to the paresis of an elevator or a depressor muscle.

Spastic Hyperphoria

It is due to an over action of one or both inferior oblique muscles.

ROLE OF REFRACTIVE ERRORS

Influence of refraction on heterophoria is as follows:

Esophoria may result from a demand for:

1. Increased accommodation, as in:
   a. Bilateral superable hypermetropia or
   b. Superable hypermetropia of the eye which sees better at all distances, whatever the refraction of the other eye.
2. Increased convergence, as in bilateral congenital myopia.

   Exophoria may result form a demand for:
   a. Decreased accommodation, as in bilateral acquired myopia.
   b. Decreased convergence, as in recession of the near point in presbyopia.

Decreased accommodation of one eye and decreased convergence, as in myopic hypermetropic anisometropia, in which the dominant eye is myopic or subnormally hypermetropic.

SYMPTOMS OF HETEROPHORIA

Heterophoria can be described as fully compensated or uncompensated. In the fully compensated type of heterophoria ocular symptoms do not develop due to: (i) strong reserve neuromuscular power available to maintain the eyes in the physiological position and also (ii) strong strength of desire for a binocular vision. If however, either one or both of these factors are weak, the muscle imbalance tends to become uncompensated/decompensated and symptoms occur.

Factors predisposing towards decompensation of heterophoria are:

Bodily ill health	:	Symptoms may arise during illness.
Ocular fatigue	:	Symptoms may arise during periods of overwork.
Mental ill health	:	Symptoms may arise during periods of anxiety and worry.
Certain occupations	:	Jobs which entail prolonged ocular activity whether it be for close work as in clerks, typists or for distance as in night drivers.
Advancing age	:	At the less easily adaptable age of middle life, symptom may begin to arise.

Classified the symptoms of heterophoria into four main types:

1. ***Symptoms due to muscular fatigue (caused by the continuous use of the reserve neuromuscular power). These are:***

- Headaches (especially occurring during or following prolonged use of eyes as in reading, watching TV/film, etc.)
- Difficulty in changing the focus for near objects after looking at a distance and *vice versa*.

Photophobia (sometimes) occurring in bright light, not relieved by wearing dark glasses but getting relieved by closing one eye.

2. ***Symptoms due to failure to maintain constant binocular vision:***

a. Blurring of print/running together of words while reading.
b. Intermittent diplopia — occur under conditions of fatigue or general debility. Horizontal diplopia particularly when viewing distant objects suggest esophoria, when viewing near objects suggest exophoria. Vertical diplopia suggests hyperphoria. Sometimes intermittent squint without diplopia is usually noticed by patient's friends. It is seen in some cases of exophoria associated with intermittent divergent squint. Intermittent convergent squint occurs in some cases of esophoria.

3. ***Symptoms due to defective postural sensation:*** Transmitted from the ocular muscles as a result of alteration of muscle tonus: like difficulty in judging the position of moving objects, difficulty in judgment in carrying out precision tool work and difficulty in estimating distances from the ground.

4. ***Symptoms due to defective stereoscopic vision*:** Ocular fatigue and difficulty in maintaining stereopsis may be met within those whose job entails the use of a stereoscope, binocular microscope. Defective stereopsis may also account for difficulties in visual judgment whose ocular muscle balance is otherwise normal.

Patients always relate the symptoms to use of their eyes and to so-called eye strain. Complaints range from redness and a feeling of heaviness, dryness and soreness of the eyes to pain in and around the eyes, frontal and occipital headaches and even gastric symptoms and nervous exhaustions. The eyes are easily fatigued and such patients often have an eversion to reading and studying. Typically these complaints tend to be less severe or disappear altogether when patients do not use their eyes in close work. Close work also is easier when the patient is rested or when one eye is closed.

Asthenopic symptoms are less frequent in distant vision than in near vision because there is less strain on the sensorimotor system. They noted that maintenance of proper alignment of the eyes may represent a considerable strain on the sensorimotor system of the eyes. Hence asthenopic symptoms tend to occur during the last years of school or college or in professional work requiring prolonged closed application, but rarely if ever in preschool children.

Exophoria

Symptoms arising due to exophoria are typically those common to all types of heterophoria. That the constant movements of converging of the eyes when moving from one end of one line to the beginning of the next and abdicative movements at the beginning of the line are undoubtedly a source of fatigue to exophorics who do much reading. That in exophorics, headaches, blurring of vision and fatigue are usually most marked during close work. Spasm of accommodation frequently occurs in an attempt to straighten the visual axes by convergence, a complete failure of fusion may supervene resulting in diplopia, or migraine, nausea and nervous prostration may force the discontinuance of the visual task.

Patients with exophoria commonly complain of eye strain, blurring of vision difficulties with prolonged periods of reading, headaches and diplopia.

Esophoria

In milder cases of esophoria symptoms are usually absent. In the more severe cases are symptoms of headache, blurring of vision and fatigue particularly evident on reading. Discomfort accompanies the use of eyes at all distances. An abnormal posture of tilting the chin downwards and head forwards is characteristic of esophoria associated with V phenomenon.

In addition to visual symptoms, reflex and psychological disturbances are often prominent in esophorics. If power of fusion is strong, a relatively large esophoria may be tolerated easily especially in cases of accommodative origin, but with considerable binocular instability the symptoms are accentuated so much so that a manifest dissociation occurs.

Unless heterophoria is intermittent, in which case the patient may be aware periodic diplopia, the symptoms in esophoria are asthenopic and related to visual demands made on the eyes. Asthenopic complaints occurring in the morning or after periods of rest are rarely caused by heterophorias. Whether esophoria becomes symptomatic or not it largely depends on the patients amplitude of fusional divergence.

Sensory Adaptation in Heterophorias

Suppression in heterophoria as a sensory adaptation may present a real obstacle to a functional cure. It is possible that suppression may then prevail to avoid foveal diplopia and fusion is maintained by peripheral retinal stimulation only. They believed that deficient stereopsis in heterophoric patients may be explained on the basis of this suppression. Usual subjective symptoms of heterophoria are in evidence—ocular pain, headache, premature fatigue on attempting close visual tasks, vertigo, nausea, generalized functional disturbances with blurring of vision, leading to temporary but irritational diplopia when the patient is tired.

Role of Hereditary

The incidence of hereditary strabismus in a strabismic population has been estimated as 30 to 70%. There are probably two types of inheritance.

1. A defect in the ectoderm, involving the nerve tissues.
2. A defect in the mesoderm involving such structures as muscles, check ligaments and facial attachments.

INVESTIGATIONS

History

a. *Visual symptoms*: Difficulty in doing near/far work blurring of vision, running of letters, intermittent diplopia/deviation, difficulty in changing focus, difficulty in judging distances from the ground, difficulty in judging position of moving objects, and difficulty in maintaining stereopsis.
b. *Ocular symptoms*: Headache, eyeache, lacrimation, tiredness of eyes, heaviness of eyes and photophobia.
c. *General symptoms*: Headache, giddiness, nausea, vomiting, mental ill health and bodily ill health.

Past history regarding any ocular trouble, wearing of glasses, previous refractive status, or general illness, etc. was elicited.

Ophthalmic Examination

a. *Visual acuity* It was tested both for near and distance, with and without glasses.
b. *Ocular examination* was done by torch light.
c. *Ocular movements*: Uniocular and binocular movements were recorded in all the cardinal nine gazes.
d. *Orthoptic investigations*: The cases were fully investigated to find out the condition of muscle balance as indicated below:

Interpupillary Distance

Cover test: The presence of heterophoria may be detected by noting that one eye deviates when it is covered, and that it makes a movement to regain binocular fixation when the cover is removed.

The cover test was carried out both for near and distance and if there was a relevant refractive error, then the test was performed both with and without the spectacle corrections. The fixation object used was a small light placed at about 1/3 meter distance and at 6 meters distance.

The findings of the cover test were recorded as follows:

The test was also repeated several times, in order to detect even a small degree of latent deviation.

Maddox rod and Maddox wing test: Heterophoria for distance was measured by Maddox rod **(Fig. 8.1)**. Heterophoria for near was measured by Maddox wing **(Fig. 8.2)**. Both these tests cause dissociation of the two eyes so that a true reading can only be obtained when the subject has got binocular vision.

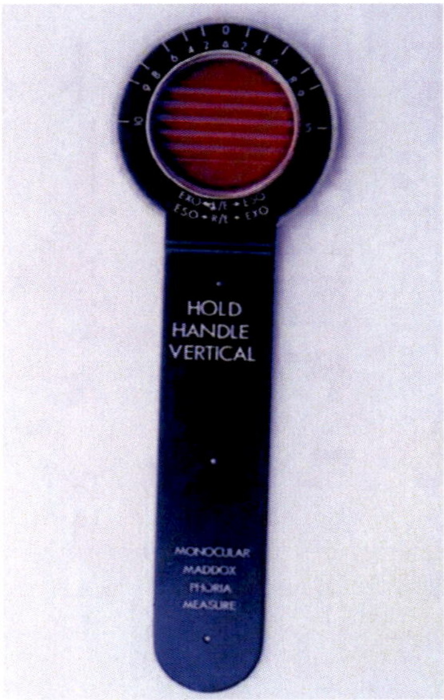

FIG. 8.1: Maddox rod

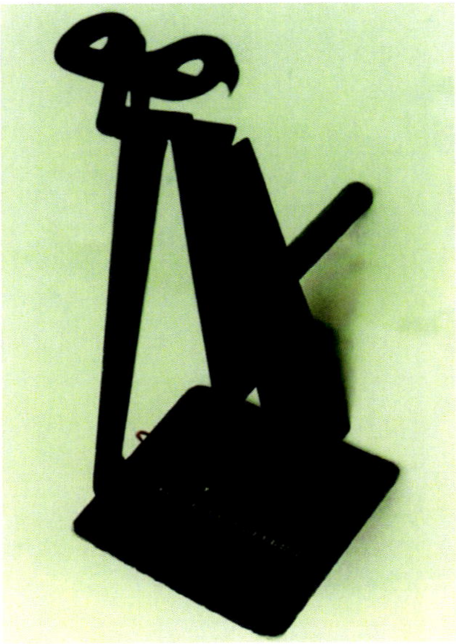

FIG. 8.2: Maddox wing

Near point of convergence: It was measured with the RAF. Near point rule **(Fig. 8.3)** which is simply a rod calibrated in centimeters, on which a card holder can slide backwards or forwards. In this holder, a card is inserted carrying a black vertical line. The proximal end of the rod was placed over the upper lip of the patient, while he fixed his eyes on the

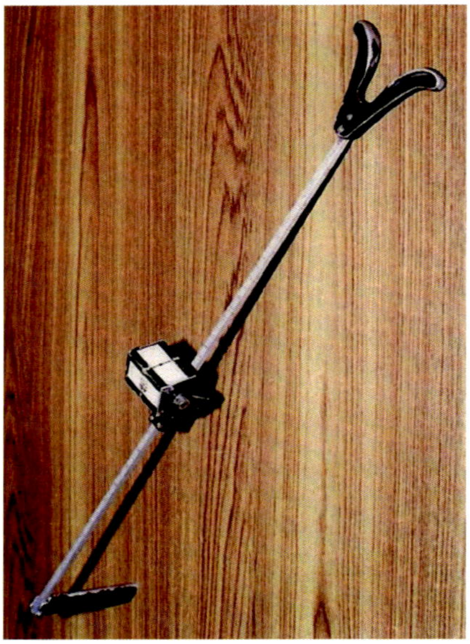

FIG. 8.3: Near point of convergence

vertical line which was slowly moved towards him until the line appeared double. The distance was read on the scale and recorded as the near point of convergence.

Worth four dot test: It was done for confirming the presence of binocular single vision.

Examination on the major amblyoscope: Before commencing examination, the instrument was adjusted for the patients height and interpupillary distance. The major amblyoscope consists of two tubes carrying illuminated slide holders which can be moved in various directions **(Fig. 8.4)**. Pairs of slides were placed in the slots provided for them. The image of these slides are dissociated and appear to be in front of the patient at infinity (6 meters). Appropriate slides were used to test for simultaneous perception, fusion angle, range of fusion and stereopsis.

Simultaneous Macular Perception

The picture used to measure simultaneous macular perception were dissimilar in size and shape such as house and joker **(Fig. 8.5)**.

Fusion

After estimating the objective and the subjective angle of fusion, the range of fusion was found out with the help of two similar slides with a

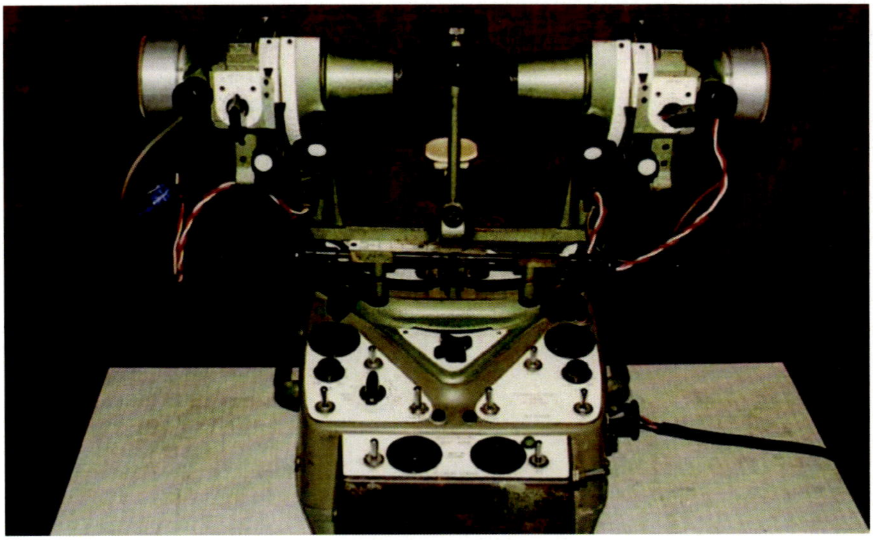

FIG. 8.4: Major amblyoscope

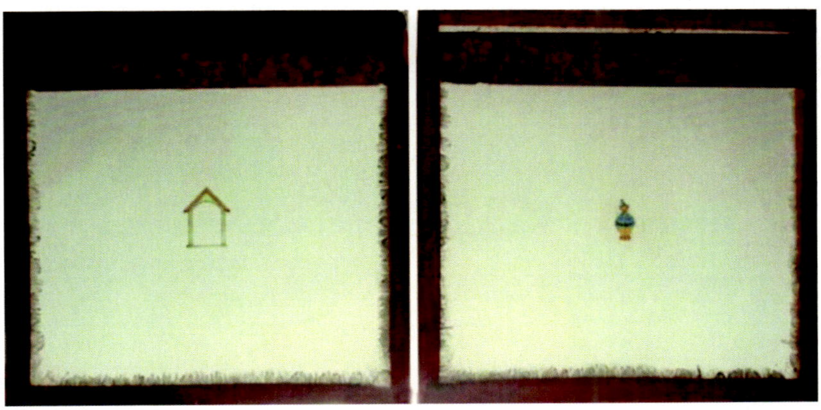

FIG. 8.5: Simultaneous macular perception

dissimilarity in each to act as a control. For example, one child and one tree in one side and second child and second tree in another slide (Fig. 8.6). Patient's ability to fuse the two images were recorded by making the patient's eyes diverge and converge with the movement of the tubes. The reading on both sides of reference point represent the fusion range.

The normal range of fusion as measured from 0° on the major amblyoscope is that of 30°-35° convergence. 5° of divergence and 3°-4° of vertical vergence.

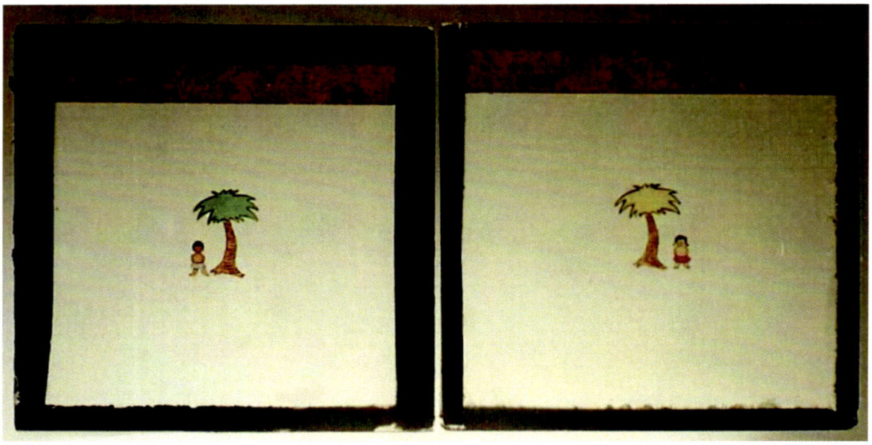

FIG. 8.6: Fusion slide

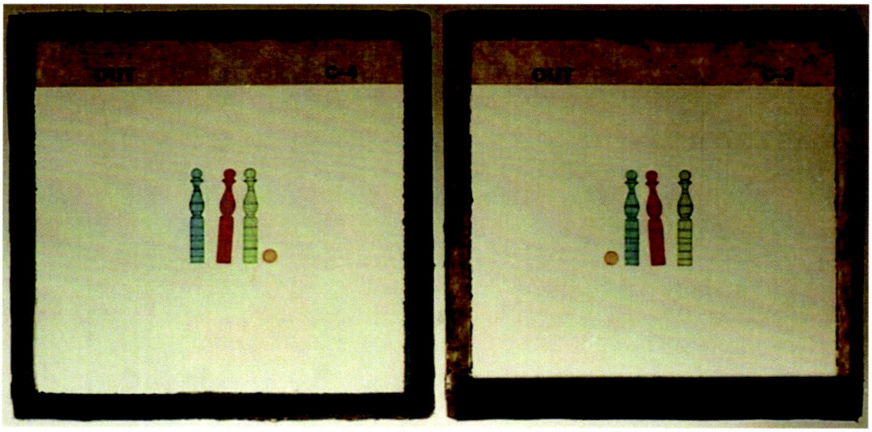

FIG. 8.7: Stereopsis

Stereopsis

Stereoscopic slides were used to find out whether the patient had Stereopsis. It was tested with the help of a slide which consisted of three wickets (Fig. 8.7). Patient was asked to indicate the direction towards which one of the three wickets was tilted. If he was able to tell correctly he was considered to have stereopsis.

Accommodative Convergence/Accommodation Ratio (AC/A Ratio)

AC/A ratio was measured on the major amblyoscope by using concave lenses of -3D in front of each eye and slides of simultaneous foveal perception (Fig. 8.8).

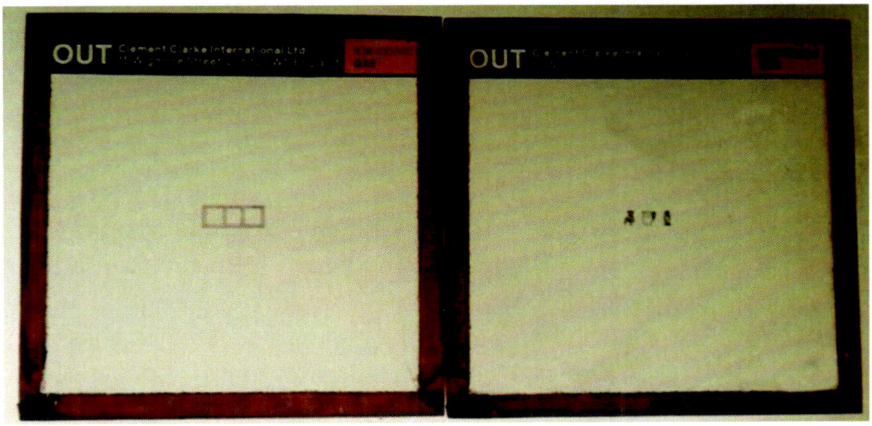

FIG. 8.8: Foveal perception slide

The patient was asked to see simultaneous foveal perception slides, wearing his spectacle correction, if any. He brought the three objects into the three squares by the movement of the side tubes, which gave the reading for subjective angle. Now, concave lenses of -3D were inserted into the lens holder and again the subjective angle was taken.

AC/A was calculated by using the following formula:

Δ_1 = subjective angle measured with the patients own vision in prism diopters.

Δ_2 = subjective angle measured with the addition of -3DS lenses in prism diopters.

D = dioptric power of the concave lens used.

Refraction

Retinoscopy was done by plane mirror under mydriasis. In young children, strong cycloplegic like homatropine 2% was used, while in adults 1% cyclopentolate was used.

Acceptance: Postmydriatic test was done after the effect of the drug had worn off till the best corrected visual acuity was achieved.

TREATMENT OF HETEROPHORIA

Orthoptic Treatment

A number of patients who has a weak binocular vision or suppression of the more ametropic eye on effort was make to build binocular vision with orthoptic exercises as follows:

1. *Antisuppression exercises*: On cherioscope, chasing and flashing exercises on major amblyoscope were with the use of simultaneous macular perception slides. It was given in those cases who has complete or partial suppression of more ametropic eye with a view to provide stimulus to the suppressed eye. The exercises were given 10 to 15 times daily.
2. *Fusion exercises*: A fusion exercises on major amblyoscope: Fusion exercises were given on major amblyoscope with the fusion slides. Fusion range could be increased by gradually converging both the tubes of major amblyoscope till the fusion breaks. Exercises were given daily or on alternate days for 10 to 15 minutes depending on the rolerance and convenience of the patients.

   When difficulty is experienced accommodation may be induced by inserting –3D sph. In the lens carriers. Patients should be taught to relax accommodation while adducting, i.e. keeping the pictures clear to 20° to 25°. Abduction should be performed without any sine of spasm. As a final exercises, when adduction to 50°C is achieved with fusion picture and voluntary adduction with simultaneous perception pictures should be attained. It should on no account be given when adduction is unsteady with fusion pictures, as it is difficult exercise to perform smoothly.

   i. *Home exercises*: Home exercises comprising of convergence to near point (Pencil to nose exercise) and reorganization of physiological diplopia for near and distance was explained to the patient. Patients were instructed to do exercises almost two to three times daily for 10 to 15 minutes.
   ii. *Fusion exercises on diploscope*: It is based on physiological diplopia and require simultaneous use of the eyes and provides convergence to the eyes.
   iii. *Physiological diplopia with pencil and distant light.*
3. Ex. diploscope exercise
4. Exercise on Remy separator
5. Exercise with the help of stereogram cards
6. Occlusion to induce use of eye with marked suppression.

Great care must be taken if this is undertaken and the occluder is best worn for reading, cinema, etc. not worn walking about. Treatment of all types of heterophoria is basically the same.

Prisms: Prisms to correct esophoria on exophoria are not advised. Patients who are unable to attend for treatment, who are unfit or too old may get relief from symptoms with prisms. Prism to correct a vertical deviation are often necessary.

Operation

Operation is necessary:

a. If the deviation is becoming manifest.
b. If the deviation is large and the patient is unable to maintain comfortable ocular vision.

Patient, should be totally occluded for a short period before the operation into manifest the full deviation.

Hyperphoria

Small degrees of hyperphoria give rise to symptoms. Large degrees are usually suppressed and do not give rise to symptoms.

Patients with hyperphoria lose their fusion range which may be the cause of symptoms. So lateral muscles range need attention.

It is rarely possible to reduce or compensate for a hyperphoria with orthoptic treatment.

Prisms should be used to compensate the vertical deviation.

Large hyperphoria are usually paretic in origin and often require surgery to compensate for the deviation.

Basic Orthoptic Treatment

a. Clip-on vertical prisms where necessary.
b. Make sure that the fusion range and muscle control is within normal limits.

Cyclophoria

Never seen unless associated with a paralysis of an elevator or depressor muscle, (External rectus palsy slight cyclo on extreme).

1. In traumatic cases, if treated early, it will disappear as the range of fusion increases and the patient obtains binocular single vision (BSV) with the help of prisms.
2. In cases of diplopia of long standing, cyclophoria cannot be overcome except by surgical treatment.
3. Small degrees often appear with an aphakia who has diplopia when wearing a contact lens. If the contact lens is given reasonably soon after operation, the cyclophoria can be overcome.

Convergence Insufficiency

It can be defined as a condition in which the parallel movements of the eyes are normal but the associated movement of simultaneous contraction of medial rectus muscles is reduced in power, normal near point of convergence is between 6–10 cm. Even it may be a normal limit but there may be inability to maintain convergence without undue effort which constitutes some degree of convergence insufficiency.

Convergence insufficiency may exist as a separate entity or may exist in association with exophoria or esophoria, etc.

There are seven types of convergence insufficiency:
1. Primary idiopathic
2. Secondary to primary divergent strabismus (divergence excess type)
3. Secondary to a vertical muscle defect
4. Convergence insufficiency due to refractive error
5. Systemic convergence insufficiency (poor general health)
6. Convergence insufficiency associated with presbyopia
7. Surgically induced convergence insufficiency.

General Physical Causes

Intoxications and diseases of endocrine glands (Moebius sign or convergence insufficiency in exophthalmos).

Psychologic causes are anxiety, neurosis.

The symptoms are those of visual fatigue in general. When convergence insufficiency alone is involved, the symptoms appear in near work after some time, and disappear quickly with rest.

Examination shows, orthophoria for distance and exophoria for near. During the effort of convergence, the pupil may remain in relative mydriasis.

In pure convergence insufficiency, which is rather rare, there will be orthophoria to 30 cm, and only from this point can the insufficiency be demonstrated.

Treatment

To treat convergence insufficiency, additional fusional convergence should be developed with the appropriate exercises.

Fusional convergence can be developed by teaching the patient to converge on objects progressively closer to his eyes while maintaining binocular vision.

The patient is taught to constantly check that he is using both eyes in any fusional convergence training. To check on the use of both eyes, the patient must have some clue. For example, if the patient tries to bring the tip of the pencil closer and closer to his nose, a different color pencil should be held further away. The image of the pencil held further away will fall on noncorresponding retinal points, and the patient will see two images of the distant pencil.

The patient attempts to bring one pencil closer to his nose while seeing two images of the pencil held farther away. He sees only one image of the nearer pencil if he is aligning his foveas because the images of the near pencil strike corresponding foveal areas on the retina.

The two pencil fusional convergence exercise is easy to teach to most patients. The patient is instructed to bring the pencil progressively closer to him and try to see the point singly while seeing two of the pencils held farther away. The single point may be blurred because the limit of accommodative convergence has been exceeded and only fusional convergence is being used. Practice in the above would be expected to increase the patient's fusional convergence.

a. *Convergence paralysis*: In this condition the patient gets diplopia on placing even the smallest power of prism before the eye. On the contrary the patient with convergence insufficiency does tolerate prisms to the extent permitted by the amount of convergence present.

Secondly, the patient will demonstrate constriction of pupil on attempted convergence. In the case of convergence insufficiency the pupillary constriction will accompany convergence movement but it will dilate as soon as the limits of convergence is crossed and the eyes diverge.

b. *Accommodative effort syndrome*: The patients of convergence insufficiency are usually associated with an exophoria for near, while in case of accommodative effort syndrome no heterophorias are associated.

When a lens of -3D is placed before the eye in a case of convergence insufficiency, there is an enhancement of convergence, while under similar circumstances the case of accommodative effort syndrome will demonstrate a tropia.

Placing of plus lenses before the eye reduces convergence by on account of relaxation of the accommodative convergence, while the accommodation is helped in cases of accommodative effort syndrome.

Treatment

It is indicated in children with poor fusional reserve and a child starts having intermittent exotropia. In adults the treatment is indicated when the symptoms are present. It consists of:

Optical Treatment

Any refractive error present is corrected after a meticulous refraction. While a full correction is prescribed for myopes, a slight under correction is made in hypermetropes. This strategy helps to improve the accommodational convergence.

Orthoptic Treatment

Orthoptic treatment is primarily aimed at improving the amplitude of convergence. Same set of exercises are done as in the case of treating exophoria, and consist of:

A. *Improving near point of convergence,* which include:

i. *Advancement exercises*: In this exercise the patient is asked to hold an object (preferably with some minute details) some distance away from his nose, and then gradually bring it closer to the nose until he sees it double. At this point he is told to withdraw the object slightly away till it becomes single again. This position is to be maintained for few moments following which the exercise process is repeated several times. Over a period of time the patient should be able to bring and keep the object almost to the tip of his nose, maintaining a binocular single vision (i.e. single object is being seen) all the time.

ii. *Jump convergence exercise*: This, in fact is an extension of advancement exercise, and should be undertaken after a successful completion of the latter. It trains the patient to maintain binocular single vision under the circumstances when a rapid change in the amount of convergence is required. Two objects are used for this exercise, one being placed at a distance of 6 meters, and the other at 33 cm away front of the patient. The patient is then asked to look at the two objects alternately. Gradually, the distance of the near object is brought closer or about 5 cm away from the nose, while maintaining a binocular single vision all the timer though the near object may look blurred.

This exercise can also be done with the help of prisms by asking the patient to fix at a near object and then placing a 10D prism with base out in front of one eye. The patient is then encouraged to maintain single vision for which he has to converge. Gradually, the demand for more and more convergences brought about by a granual increase in the power of the prism until the patient can converge to maintain single vision with prism of 40D.

B. *Improving amplitude of fusional convergence*: The following exercises may be undertaken to improve the amplitude of fusional convergence:

i. *Exercises with prisms*: Prisms of increasing power, with base out, are placed before the patient's eye while he is fixing at a near object. He is encouraged to maintain single vision when the prism's is being increased. Use of a prism bar for this purpose is more appropriate.

ii. *Exercises on synoptophore*: The patient is asked to fuse the two stereoscopic slides and then the tubes are slowly converged until he fusion is broken as evidenced by the loss of stereopsis. The procedure is repeated again and again for about five minutes on weekly basis. In the intervening period home exercises are continued.

iii. *Physiological diplopia exercise*: This is performed with help of a card. Before starting the procedure the patient is first made to appreciate physiological diplopia. The stereogram is held at arm's length in front of the patient and he is asked to fix at the picture. At this point a pencil is placed midway between the card and the patient.

iv. *Exercise on diploscope:* Exercises for voluntary convergence—This is a very useful exercise that needs the cooperation of an intelligent patient who is asked to fix at a distant object, preferably a small source of light. At this stage another object say a pencil or a finger is interposed and placed in front of the patient at about an arm's length. The patient is now asked to fix his gaze at the pencil and is encouraged to appreciate doubling of the distant fixation object, which results as the pencil is being fixed (physiological diplopia). The pencil is then removed from the field of vision and the patient is asked to keep on with seeing double images of the distant object. This procedure may be repeated several times. In due course of time the patient is trained to see double images of the distant object, even without the introduction of the pencil.

Prism Treatment or Prismotherapy

Prism treatment or prismotherapy is reserved for cases not responding favorably to the orthoptic treatment. Base in prisms are corporated in the correcting glasses. In general, prescription of prisms is avoided in children.

Surgical Treatment

Operative interference should be made as the 1st alternative when all other forms of treatment fail to relieve the symptoms. A unilateral or bilateral resection of the medial rectus muscle may be undertaken.

Convergence Paralysis

As already described it is the result of some intracranial lesions involving the midbrain and the III N nucleus. The diagnostic features are:
- Sudden onset
- Exotropia and crossed diplopia on attempted convergence.

Normal Adduction

- Usually normal accommodation.
- Preservation of miosis and accommodation on attempted convergence.
- Evidence of intracranial lesion.

Diplopia caused by the weak base out prism (while a case or convergence deficiency tolerates base out prisms to a certain extent).

Treatment: Appropriate prisms are prescribed for near vision. If binocular single vision cannot be achieved, occlusion of one eye be done while doing near work. Surgical interference is not indicated.

Convergence Spasm

It is rare anomaly of convergence which is mostly of functional nature. Rarely it may be caused by some intracranial disease. It is characterized by:
- Intermittent attacks of extreme convergence resembling a bilateral palsy of VI N
- Intermittent homonymous diplopia
- Blurring of vision caused by associated spasm of accommodation
- Miotic pupils, as a part of the near reflex
- Myopia upto 6D, induced by the spasm of accommodation.

Treatment

Most of the cases need psychiatric treatment, after the possibility of an intracranial has been excluded. The palliative measures may be adopted in the form of prolonged atropinization or occlusion of one eye as an alternative.

9 *Pseudostrabismus*

PSEUDOESOTROPIA

Epicanthus—It is a bilateral condition, which may be associated with ptosis. A more or less vertical fold of skin runs from the root of the nose to the inner end of the lower eyelid, covering the medical canthus and the caruncle.

If such folds are prominent they produce or apparent convergent strabismus.

PSEUDODIVERGENT STRABISMUS

An apparent divergent strabismus may be produced by one or more of the following factors:

1. A large positive angle alpha
2. A wide interpupillary distance
3. Exophthalmos
4. A wide palpebral fissure.

If binocular single vision is present, the parents should reassured that there is no actual deviation.

i. If the orbits are set wide apart producing a wide interpupillary distance, exophoria is common. If orbits are set close together, resulting in narrow interpupillary distance, esophoria is common.
ii. If there is exophthalmos (as seen in hyperthyroidism), there will be some displacement of the eyeball out made as well as forwards, exophoria usually occurs. The presence of an undue narrowing of the lateral canth causes an apparent divergent squint because of the reduced amount of the eyeball which is visible on the lateral side of each canthus.
iii. The presence of abnormally large angle alpha.

The presence of a large positive (or nasal) angle alpha may produce an apparent divergent strabismus.

In the average normal eye the visual axis does not coincide with the optic axis (or midpupillary line) but cuts the corneal to the nasal side of the latter. (This is because the fovea is situated slightly downwards and to the temporal side of the point at which the optic axis cuts the ratina) this means that there is a small angle between the optic axis and visual axis. This angle, which rarely exceeds 5° to 7° is known as angle alpha. When visual axis cuts the cornea on the nasal side of the optic axis, it is said to be positive angle alpha and when visual axis cuts the cornea on the temporal side, it is side to be negative angle alpha. For purpose of measurement of angle alpha on major amblyoscope, we use a special slide consisting of row of numbers and letters at intervals of one degree. This slide is placed in front of the eye under observation. The patient should be told to look at the '0'. If the corneal reflection in observed to be to the nasal side of the pupil the angle alpha is positive, if it is to the temporal side the angle alpha is negative. Then we ask the patient to look at each of the numbers or letters in turn, until the reflection on the cornea is observed to be central. This procedure is then repeated using the slide before the other eye and in this way we can record positive and negative angle alpha.

PSEUDOHYPERTROPIA

If one orbit is slightly higher than the other due to a symmetry of the skull, then are appearance of vertical strabismus may result. Facial asymmetrics or orbital tumors, the mass can displace the globe vertically and may stimulate vertical ocular deviation.

10 Manifest and Concomitant Squints

A. MANIFEST SQUINT

CLASSIFICATION OF SQUINT

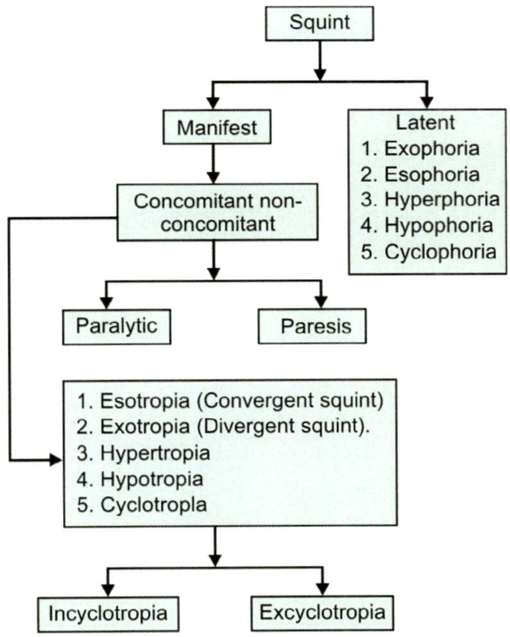

B. CONCOMITANT SQUINT

Normally, both eyes are maintained at the point of fixation under various central and peripheral influences. In ordinary activity both eyes are directed at the point of fixation together. If the position of fixation is not maintained so that one eye gets deviated, the condition of heterotropia or manifest squint arises.

The manifest squint may be either concomitant or incomitant. The word concomitant is derived from Latin 'concomitor' meaning 'I attend, I accompany'. In fact, in a concomitant squint the deviation remains the same, or approximately so, in all positions of the gazes. The eyes thus move together in coordination retaining the abnormal relationship between them with all ocular movements.

According to Duke Elder, concomitant squint is of two types — primary and secondary. Primary concomitant squint develops due to obstacle in sensory or afferent pathway of binocular vision so that eyes are dissociated but coordinated by postural reflexes which retains the motor axis unimpaired. It is a bilateral condition, the deviation being shared equally between two eyes. When one eye fixes the deviation of both becomes manifest in the other eye. In secondary concomitant squint, there is a peripheral muscular basis; it follows secondarily upon the incomitant squint.

Classification

The concomitant squint is clinically classified based on different parameters.

1. Depending upon the direction of deviation:
   Esotropia—the deviating eye turns inwards
   Exotropia—the deviating eye turns outwards
   Hypertropia—the deviating eye turns upwards
   Hypotropia—the deviating eye turns downwards
   Cyclotropia—torsional defect where the deviation takes the form of a rotation round the fixation axis.
2. Depending upon the constant or intermittent presence of the deviation: Constant and intermittent types.
3. Depending upon the fixation preference:
   Uniocular squint—affects one eye so that the other eye is preferred for fixation.

Alternating squint—alternate involvement of the eyes and no obvious preference for fixing with either eye.

4. Depending upon the time of onset:
   Congenital squint—deviation noticed in early months of life.
   Infantile squint—deviation noticed before 1 year of age.
   Acquired squint—deviation noticed after 2 years of age. In primary acquired squint no definite cause can be found and it is acute in onset. In secondary type, the deviation arises from known cause such as disease of the eyes or trauma or operation. Consecutive cases are the result of change in the nature of squint—either spontaneous or occurring after attempted squint surgery.
5. Depending upon the fusional and accommodative vergence: Convergence weakness or excess, divergence weakness or excess, basic types; typical accommodative, partially accommodative, hypo-accommodative, nonaccommodative types.

Periodic squint is a special type as reported by Duke-Elder, which differs in degree depending on far or near fixation. If the squint is greater for near, it is called directly periodic; if greater for distance, inversely periodic.

Cyclic squint—Cyclic squint is another special type in which the squint appears and disappears in a rhythmic manner, most frequently at 48 hours intervals.

Convergent concomitant squint or esotropia may be primary, secondary due to loss of vision or consecutive following overcorrection of exotropia by surgery.

According to Duke-Elder there are three main forms of primary esotropia.

1. Esotropia of the convergence excess type in which the deviation is significantly greater for near.
   a. Accommodative esotropia
      i. Typical accommodative esotropia in which the deviation is cured by correction of the underlying hypermetropia.
      ii. Atypical accommodative esotropia with no significant refractive error. It may be either hypoaccommodative or hyper-accommodative with high AC/A ratio.
      iii. Partially accommodative esotropia—the commonest accommodative squint where uncorrected hypermetropia is partly responsible for the deviation.

b. Tonic esotropia

c. Esotropia with congenital myopia.

2. Esotropia of the divergence weakness type in which the deviation is greater for distance.
3. Esotropia of the basic type in which the deviation is almost same in distance and near.

A few other forms of esotropia are:

4. Essential (infantile) esotropia—characterized by early onset, large deviation, no significant refractive error and frequent association of vertical component.
5. Acute concomitant esotropia.
6. Cyclic esotropia.
7. Microtropia—characterized by small deviation, amblyopia, eccentric fixation with central scotoma and harmonious retinal correspondence.

Among the causes of primary concomitant convergent squint few important ones are excess use of accommodation in hypermetropia, uncompensated esophoria, congenital myopia and anatomical conditions like asymmetry of orbits, etc. There is a special form of convergent squint which may be associated with the following:

1. *Congenital myopia:* Near object seen clearly, but distant objects cannot be seen and so all distant objects appear blurred to him so there is no initiative to keep the eyes straight and they converge.
2. *Other causes:*
   i. Corneal opacity
   ii. Lenticular opacity
   iii. Chorioretinal atrophy
   iv. Optic atrophy
   v. Pseudoglioma
   vi. Retinoblastoma
3. *Consecutive convergent squint:* Over correction of divergent squint can lead to consecutive convergent squint.
4. *Ocular palsy*: Primary vertical concomitant squint is rare. Most of the vertical components are associated with primarily horizontal concomitant squint cases, usually esotropias. The etiology of truly concomitant vertical deviations of magnitude rarely exceding few prism diopters is not clear. There can be A-V pattern, overaction of inferior obliques and dissociated vertical deviations associated with primarily horizontal concomitant squint cases.

Etiological Causes (Duke Elder)

1. *Optical obstacles:* Preventing the formation of suitable retinal images. These are of 2 types:
   a. *Extraneous factors:* Seen in young children due to prolonged period of disease of one eye despite absence of any pathological lesions like:
      — Congenital ptosis
      — Effect of wrong spectacles
      — Seen in watch makers
      — Prolonged occlusion of an eye.
   b. *Ocular factors:* Like
      — High refractive errors
      — Anisometropia
      — Aniseikonia
      — Opacities in the ocular media
      — Damage to fovea/Parafovea as seen in congenital toxoplasmosis and congenital rubella.
2. *Sensory obstacles:* Preventing the association of corresponding retinocerebral points like
   — Disease of retina and optic disk
   — Lesions of the visual pathways.
3. *Motor obstacles:* Preventing adequate coordination of the 2 eyes. These can be of following types:
   a. *Static obstacles:*
      — Anomalies of symmetry and inclination of orbits and shape of skull as in craniofacial dysostosis where divergence in common
      — Abnormalities in the shape of globe as in high myopia
      — Abnormality of position of globe — as in proptosis
      — Space occupying lesions of orbits
      — Congenital abnormalities of muscles
      — Paresis of the muscles
      — Abnormalities of insertion of the muscles.
4. *Central obstacles:* Preventing the emergency of unitary binocular perception like:
   a. Faculty development of faculty of fusion

b. After the establishment of the binocular reflexes, fall in the efficiency at highest level may lead to their breakdown. The dampening of the cerebral activity is seen in:
   — Severe illness
   — Fatigue
   — Alcohol poisoning
   — Coma.
c. The factors which leads to disturbance of neural equilibrium, which in turn leading to a latent and compensated ocular imbalance to become manifest squint like in:
   — Hyperexcitability state as been in teething
   — Emotional states.

General Features

1. The deviation of the eyeball is same in all the directions of the gaze.
2. The primary deviation (deviation of the squinting eye under cover when sound eye is fixating) is equal to secondary deviation (deviation of sound eye under cover when squinting eye is fixating).
3. There is no limitation of movements of the eyeball.
4. In case of uniocular concomitant squint, the vision in the squinting eye is usually defective.
5. There is no compensatory head posture.
6. There is no abnormal projection/orientation.

Symptoms

1. Patient may complain of manifest deviation of the eye. It may be either intermittent or constant.
2. Patient may complain of diminition of vision in one or both eyes.
   i. If it is constant, there is development of suppression, which leads to amblyopia. The patient gets relief of symptoms like diplopia and headache with development of suppression.
   ii. Most of times it is associated with horizontal squint. It may be primary vertical squint with secondary horizontal or *vice versa*. The most common secondary horizontal or *vice versa*. The most common secondary vertical elements are elevation in adduction or abduction due to imbalance of vertical recti (superior and

inferior rectus) and oblique muscle (superior and inferior oblique muscles).

Cyclotropia

There are torsional defects and are extremely rare. These are usually paretic in nature and due to congenital defects.

Sequalae of Events in a Case

In a case of concomitant squint, apart from loss of binocular vision, the patient may be asymptomatic. Initially, there might be confusion, i.e. simultaneous formation of two dissimilar images of two objects, or Diplopia, i.e. simultaneous formation of two images of same object on 2-corresponding points of retina. But these symptoms disappear with the development of suppression in the squinting eye in favor of the other eye in order to avoid confusion or diplopia. The suppression may be central, i.e. inhibition of the foveal image of the squinting in order to avoid confusion or it may be peripheral, i.e. inhibition of the image from the periphery of retina or extrafoveal point in order to avoid diplopia. The suppression may be facultative in initial stages, i.e. inhibition of image when eye is deviating or obligatory, i.e. inhibition of the image irrespective of whether eye is deviated or not.

The suppression in all cases is aided by the peripheral situation of the image in the squinting eye, but the essential seat of suppression is in the brain. As the image of any object falling on noncorresponding points causes diplopia, which brain finds difficult to fuse, so it actively suppresses the image.

The prolonged suppression of image leads to permanent lowering of vision in the squinting eye, leading to a condition called *amblyopia*. In the long-standing cases, the squinting eye may or may not show any movement to take up fixation on cover test. This position of the deviation which is less than the actual deviation as called as eccentric fixation, i.e. fixation in the squinting eye is being assumed by extrafoveal point. The maximum visual acuity on the extra-foveal point is made available to the squinting eye. This is a uniocular phenomenon. While the condition where fovea of one eye corresponds with the extrafoveal point in other eye and it is called as *anomalous retinal correspondence*. It is a binocular phenomenon.

METHOD OF EXAMINATION

History

The squint itself when it was noted and how it was noted? Which eye was involved and what was the direction and type of squint? What was the mode of onset and progression? Does it present all the time in same extent? Does it vary with changing direction of gaze?

Family History

Strabismus itself is not in the strict sense directly hereditary but probably its predisposing factors such as refractive errors visual defects.

a. *Nutritional status*: Fatigue, weakness and malnutrition are important factors to aggravate concomitant squint.
b. *The possible precipitating cause*: History of any antenatal, postnatal or birth events, head injury, systemic disease particularly before or at the onset of squint were recorded. Any associated facial or systemic anomaly was recorded also.
c. *The subjective symptoms*: History of diplopia was taken. If present, uniocular or binocular, maximum in which direction of gaze, minimum in which direction of gaze and head posture were recorded. Any history of headache, eye strain, vertigo, etc. were noted also.
d. *The family history*: The family history of squint, high refractive error or any facial and systemic anomaly were noted.
e. *History of previous treatment*: Either optical or surgical or by any means were noted with emphasis on the onset and progression of the squint.

Systemic Examination (Fig. 10.1)

General physical examination and specially the neurological examination was carried out to rule out any systemic disease or neurological disorder. General appearance of the face and head was noted for any sign of skull or face deformity, malposition of orbits or trauma position of the eyelids and eyes in the orbits were checked for any abnormality—particularly ptosis, proptosis or lid lag.

Head posture was noted and abnormal head posture was recorded under following headings:

1. *Face turn :* Towards right/left/absent
2. *Head tilt:* Towards right/left/absent
3. *Chin position:* Elevated/depressed/normal.

If the head posture was nonocular, i.e. congenital torticollis or due to deafness, disorders of cervical spine or simple habit, that was noted also.

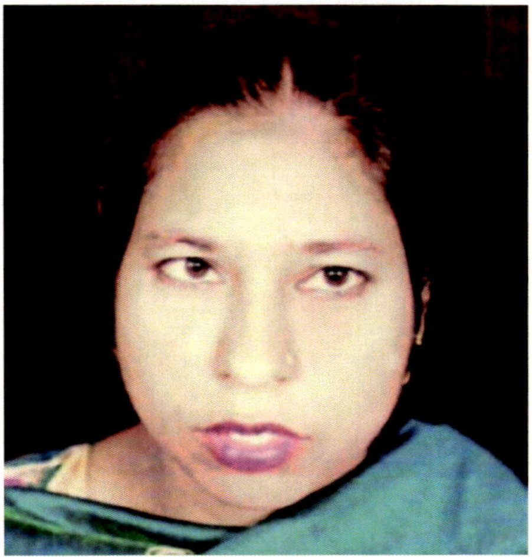

FIG. 10.1: Convergent squint

Ophthalmological Examination

Each eye was examined on torch light and slit lamp for any abnormality in the anterior segment and media. Condition of conjunctiva, cornea, anterior chamber, pupil and lens were noted. Special attention was given to pupillary light reactions—both direct and consensual.

Visual acuity in each eye with other eye occluded was tested for near and distance, without and with glass and with pinhole separately—both cortical and angular.

For distance, visual acuity was tested with an internally illuminated rotating drum having Snellen's charts placed 6 meters away from the patient **(Fig. 10.2).** So far we were testing the vision, visual acuity of infant by corneal reflex by throwing the light by torch. If reflex is central, steady and well-maintained, its means that vision visual acuity is good in infant. But now we have "Cardiff professional looking test".

Preferential Looking Test

Here was present two stimulus in the visual field

i. One stimulus is homogenous
ii. The other stimulus is having stripes.

Infant will look at a striped pattern for a greater period of time.

The method is especially suitable for infants up to four (4) months of age older infants are easily distracted.

Visual acuity is in newborn is 6/240

At 3 months 6/60

At 3 years 6/6.

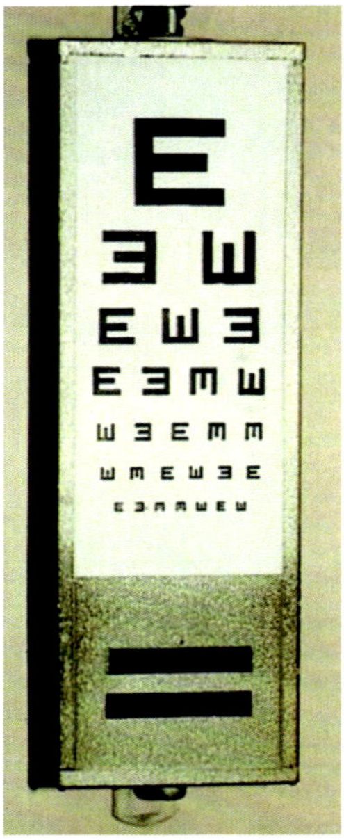

FIG. 10.2: Snellen's chart

By this test

We cannot compare the visual acuity with the acuity testing on naming the pictures for letters on Snellen's chart.

In normal children grating acuity is better than recognition acuity. The coming to visual acuity in bet 21/2-3 years. So far we were testing the visual acuity by:

1. We can test the visual acuity by Sjögren test **(Fig. 10.3)** where we shown isolated figure of a hand of asked him to match this is with isolated hands of varying size at 5 meter distance.
2. Picture snellen visual acuity test **(Fig. 10.4)**—Instead of showing symbols (letters), we present picture with which child is liking to be more familiar.
3. Dot visual acuity testing—Child is shown an illuminated box with black dots of different size printed on it. The smallest dot denotes the visuals acuity of the child.
4. Coin test—Child is asked to identity the two faces of coins of different sizes held at different distances.
5. Toy test—In this test child is shown a miniature from distance of 10ft and child is asked to name the toy (or pick the pair from the assortment).

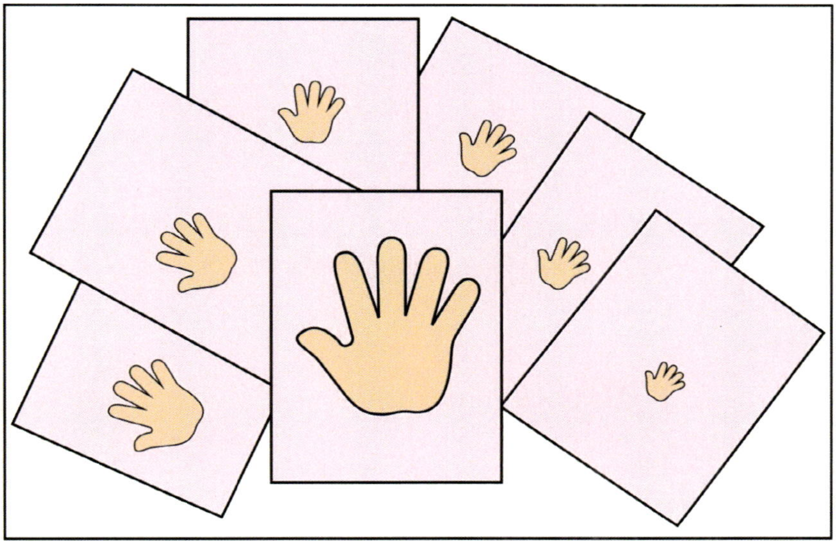

FIG. 10.3: Sjögren test

6. Marble game test—is carried out in 1 year old child. The child is asked to place marbles in hole of box. By this test, we cannot measure visual acuity of each eye, but we can compare the function of one eye when other eye is closed. The vision noted as being 'useful' or 'less useful'.
7. Optokinetic nystagmus test—In this test nystagmus is elicited by passing a succession of black and white stripes through the patient's field of vision.

   The smallest strip that can elicites an eye movement is a measure.

   The only cooperation required in this test is that the infant is: (i) awake and (ii) hold both eyes open.

This test the visual acuity is follows:

1. Newborn visual acuity 6/120
2. Visual acuity at 2 months 6/60
3. Visual acuity at 6 months 6/36
4. Visual acuity at 2 years 6/6

Contrast Sensitivity Charts

There are two charts and two scoring pads. The two charts are identical although with different letter sequences. Letters are organized in group

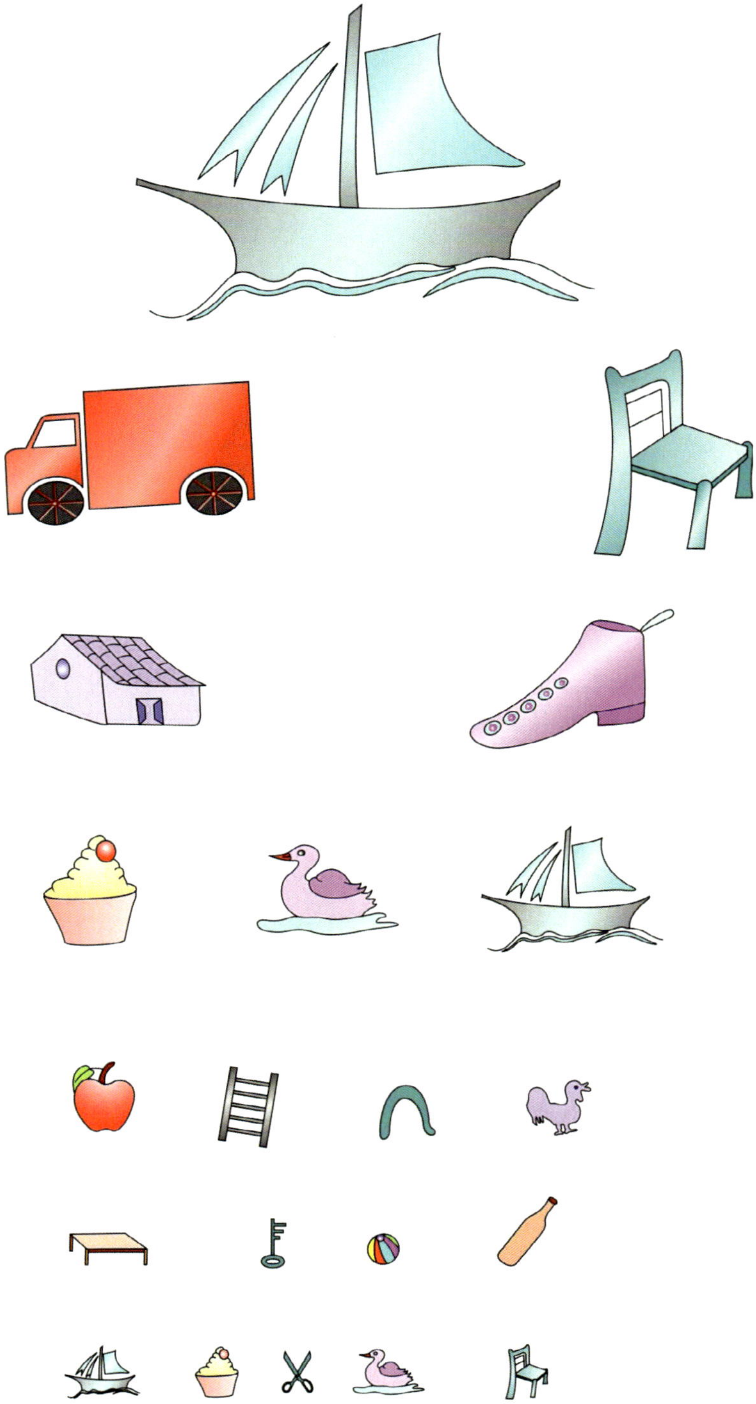

FIG. 10.4: Snellen's chart

of three. With each triplet all letters have the same contrast. The contrast decreases from one triplet to the next. The division into triplets is indicated on the scoring pad. In Snellen chart the difficulty in reading line increases from line to line but in Pelli-Robson chart the difficulty increases in the middle of each line as well. The center of chart should be approximately at the level of the patient eye. The chart should be illuminated as uniformly as possible so that luminance of the white areas is about 85ed/m^2.

We test the patient before dilating the people or applying any other drug to their eyes.

The patient should sit or stand directly in front of the chart so that the distance from the eyes to the chart is about 1 meter or 40 inches (patient should sit at 1 meter distance away from the chart and the level of the eyes should be at the center of the chart). The patient should wear their best distance correction and if necessary an addition of 0.75D. Patient should read letter from upper left hand corner and he has to read each letter on the chart. On the scoring pad underline or circle each letter correctly and strike any letter read incorrectly. Patients should be made to guess even when they believe that the letters are invisible. Do not let the patient give up too soon. You should allow several seconds for the finest letters to appear, but do not let the patient give up until he or she has guessed incorrectly 2 of 3 letters in a triplet. The reliability of the result depends on this.

Scoring pads — The patient's sensitivity is indicated by the faintest triplet for which 2 of the 3 letters are named correctly.

The patient should be tested three times. Test each eye separately and both eyes together. When you test one eye, the other eye is covered. The three measurements should take no more than 8 minutes in all.

Binocular Log contrast sensitivity is normally 0.15 higher than monocular.

The chart's plastic substrate and special ink were chosen for their great stability and contrast clarity.

The chart should not be touched by fingertips. If necessary, wipe the chart gently with soft cloth using a highly diluted solution of mild soap or detergent (e.g. lvory liquid) in water then rinse with clean water. Avoid exposure to direct sunlight or any UV light source. To prolong the life of the chart it is suggested that the chart is tuned to face the wall when not in use.

There is expiry date printed on each chart at manufacture. In this chart letters all uniformly large and they fade out towards the bottom of the chart. The top line has high contrast letters black or white. The letter below there in grey and more difficult to see, very much like looking through fog or dirty glasses.

Try to read as many letters as you can. The letters at the bottom of the chart are difficult for everyone to read so do not be discouraged. The reading one letter at a time, try blinking or viewing the letter a little eccentrically, moving your head from side to side. Ask from patient Does he see something against the white background? It is round or square? Does it has corners or lines you can see? Keep trying. The whole letter may suddenly appear to you. Go ahead and guess.

Cambridge Low Contrast Gradings

This is simple and rapid screening test for contrast sensitivity. The patient with the normal visual acuity will see the chart from 6 meter distances. Patient should wear his glasses test each eye separately.

The test comprises 12 parts of plates. The first pair serves as a demonstration. Show this pair of plates to the patient and the patient has to choose the pages or which the stripes appear on top or bottom. If he cannot see the stripes, he has to guess.

The next ten pairs of plates are numeral 1–10 and form 10 test stimuli 90 show him No. 1, 2, 3, etc. in sequence. If he fails to do so, ask him to guess. As soon as examiner note the error, note it on the score sheet (the number of the test stimulus on which the error was made). Then go back four stimuli and begin a second series when error occur more a third series. Continue until four series have been presented and then repeat for the other eye, starting the first series at number 1.

Score each eye separately. For each series note the number of the stimulus on which the error occurred. This number is the score for the series. If there is no error in the series the score is II.

E-cut Out Test (Fig. 10.5)

E test types were used as it was recognized by illiterate persons as well as young children. It consists of a series of the letter E of diminishing size downwards rotated in different directions. The patient was asked in which direction the limbs of a particular E as pointed were open. As per the standard Snellen's chart principle, the top E is so constructed that if viewed at a distance of 60 meters, it subtends an angle of 5 minutes

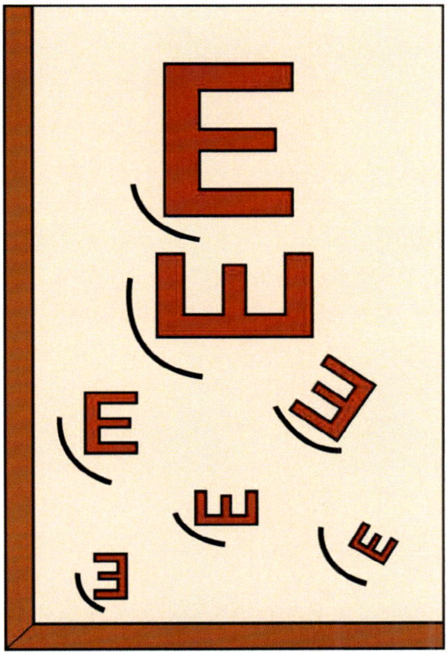

FIG. 10.5: E-cut out test

and each constituent limb subtends an angle of 1 minute at the nodal point of the viewer's eye. In order to appreciate the standard limit of 1 minute. Thus the top line can be 'read' from 60 meters, and the next ones from 36, 24, 18, 12, 9, and 5 meters respectively. The results of the test were expressed as a fraction—the numerator is the distance between the patient and the chart (usually 6 meters), the denominator is the line he could just appreciate correctly.

For near vision the Jaeger's near chart was used at 33 cm. Distance. After noting visual acuity in each eye, binocular visual acuity was measured also, keeping both eyes open in the same manner for distance and near—first with glass and then without glass.

Orthoptic Examination

Cardiff Acuity Test

Cardiff acuity test done:

1. Toddlers aged 1 to 3 years
2. Older children
3. Adults with intellectual impairment and in cases of strike or head injury
4. Malingering.

The principle of the target design is that of the vanishing optotype. The targets are drawn with a white band bordered by two bands, each one is half the thickness of the white band. All on a neutral background. If the target lies beyond the visual acuity of the child, it merges with the grey background and becomes simply invisible. Thus resolution, detection and recognition acuity threshold are all brought together. The targets used are picture, but decreasing in width of white and black bands. The narrowest white band for which the target is visible. The principle of the test is that of preferential looking are infant will choose to look towards a target, rather than towards a plain stimulus. In Cardiff test, each target is positioned either in the top half or in the bottom. Half of the card.

If the target is visible, the child will look toward sit and the examiner watch the child's eye movements.

An important feature of the preferential looking technique is that the examiner should not know in advance the position of target.

For any given target width, if examiner estimates the position correctly on two consecutive occasions, the target is assumed to be visible to the child. If the examiner is unable to make a judgment from the child's responses, then target is assumed to be beyond the child's acuity limit.

In Cardiff test, we present two cards to the child.

The target is positioned up and down so that the eye movements are easier to discriminate in cases of congenital nystagmus. The child is seated at one meter distance from the target at this distance the examiner can appreciate eye movement of the child.

This test can done at 50 cm. At this distance visual acuity is 6/120 to 6/12.

Procedure—for each visual acuity level shuffle the three cards and begin with widest target (lowest acuity) present the first card at the child's eye level. In order to draw, child attention talk about the picture, or encourage the child to point to the picture.

We can establish the visual acuity by child eye movement by estimating the position top/bottom of the target. Once you make your decision, present the second card to confirm your decision. If two correct estimates are made, proceed to the next level. If incorrect estimate is made return to the next larger target and repeat the test.

Shuffle the card between each presentation. The end point can then be taken at the highest level at which at least two out of the three cards are scored correctly. The calibration for the cards it given in table, which presents acuity levels for two distances, in both Log MAR and equivalent smaller acuity.

Cardiff preferential looking tests tend to give a higher acuity than a visual acuity on Snellen chart because the child is target and not to identify it.

Cardiff test is carried out at a near distance. Test the visual acuity with glasses, if there is any reflective error. In malingering the patient is not aware of their eye movements and will look consistently at the target even while visiting that they cannot see it.

Ductions

The test was performed at near. Each eye was covered in turn while the other eye fixated spot light held at 33 cm. and was moved in all cardinal directions of gaze. Any overaction or underaction in any direction was noted. Presence of nystagmoid movements were checked if any, particularly in full duction.

Versions: Carried out in similar manner keeping both eye uncovered to detect any underaction of one muscle with or without overaction of its antagonist and contralateral synergist, up shoot or down shoot of any eye in horizontal versions, retraction of the globe and narrowing of palpebral fissure in any direction of gaze.

Diplopia in any position of binocular gaze was noted if stated by the patient on enquiry.

Cover Test (Figs 10.6A and B)

For near the test was performed with and without glasses with a sharp object of fixation such as a spot sized small light situated at a distance of 33 cm. from the patient. The patient was asked to fixate the object and one eye was covered. Any movement in the uncovered eye was noted. An inward movement meant exotropia, outward movement esotropia, upward movement hypotropia and downward movement hypertropia of the uncovered eye. At times combination of horizontal and vertical movements were also detected indicating the presence of both horizontal and vertical squint. The test was repeated covering the other eye and looking for movement of the now uncovered eye for any manifest squint of this eye. In unilateral squint the sound eye took fixation whenever it was uncovered. In alternating squint the fixation was retained by the uncovered eye irrespective of which eye was covered.

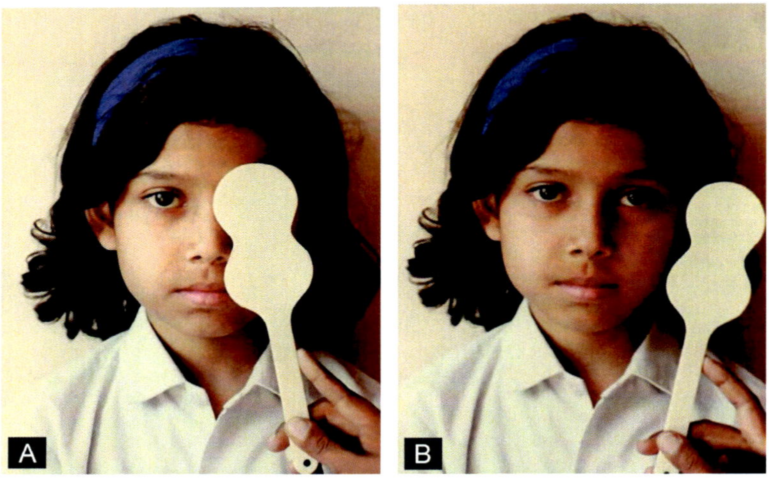

FIGS 10.6A AND B: Cover test

If no movement was detected on covering each eye in turn then alternate cover test was done—dissociating the fusion reflex by putting the cover in one eye for some time and then rapidly alternating the cover in the eyes never allowing the fusion reflex to re-establish. Movement in this test means heterophoria. If alternate cover test is done in a case of manifest unilateral squint and there is equal movement of each eye it indicates the concomitant nature of the squint (Figs 10.7 and 10.8).

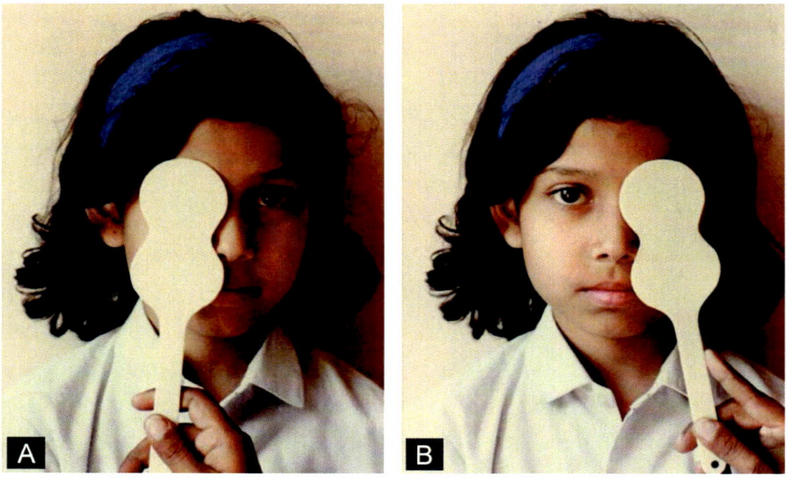

FIGS 10.7A AND B: Cover shifted to other eye and alternate cover test

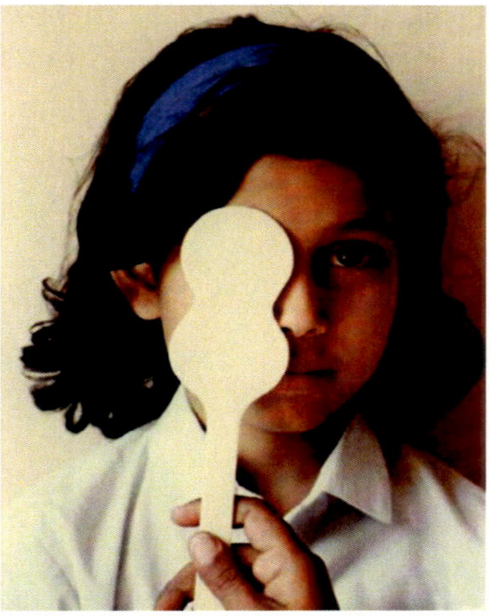

FIG. 10.8: Alternate cover test

Initially, the cover test was done in primary gaze and later it was repeated in all the main positions of conjugate gaze.

For distance: The whole test was repeated for distance, the patient being seated at a distance of 6 meters from the spot light.

The cover test provided following informations:

1. Whether there was deviation of any or not.
2. Type of the deviation—concomitant or incomitant.
3. Direction of deviation—eso/exo, hyper/hypo, incyclo/excyclo deviation.
4. Whether the deviation was constant or intermittent.
5. Whether the deviation was unilateral or alternating.
6. Approximate size of the deviation—slight, moderate or marked.
7. Primary deviation *vis-à-vis* secondary deviation.
8. Rough estimation regarding vision in case of children—get annoyed or start crying if fixing eye is occluded.
9. Presence of latent nystagmus, if any.

Fallacy of cover test; inconclusive in cases of microtropia, where there is eccentric fixation and when the patient is uncooperative.

Angle of Deviation (Fig. 10.9)

Hirschberg's Method

A rough estimation of the angle of squint was done by Hirschberg's test. A spot light was held 33 cm in front of the patient's face and he was

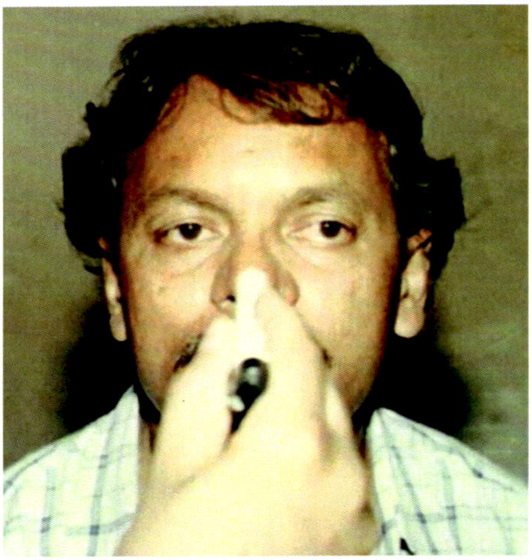

FIG. 10.9: Hirschberg's method

asked to look directly at the light. The position of the corneal reflection on the squinting eye was then noted, the observer being directly behind the light. If the reflection was situated on the nasal side of the cornea the squint was divergent, if on the temporal side the squint was convergent. Each mm. of displacement of the reflection from the center of the cornea of the squinting eye equals to 7° of arc. In general terms, if the reflection was on the margin of the pupil the deviation was 12°–15°; if on the limbus 45° and if halfway between 25°.

Prism Bar Cover Test (Fig. 10.10)

This is an objective test to measure either latent or manifest deviations. The patient was seated in front of a fixation light placed at 6 metres (for distance) or 33 cm (for near). The patient was asked to look straight at the light and alternate cover test was performed to note the movement of the eyes to take fixation when uncovered. The movement was then neutralized by the use of prisms of increasing strength incorporated in a prism bar (base in the direction of movement of the nonfixing eye, i.e. in the direction opposite to the deviation). The strength of the prism required to eliminate the movements was the amount of deviation as revealed.

The test was done both for near and distance with each eye fixing in turn, in order to exclude the presence of any incomitant element (larger secondary deviation than primary deviation).

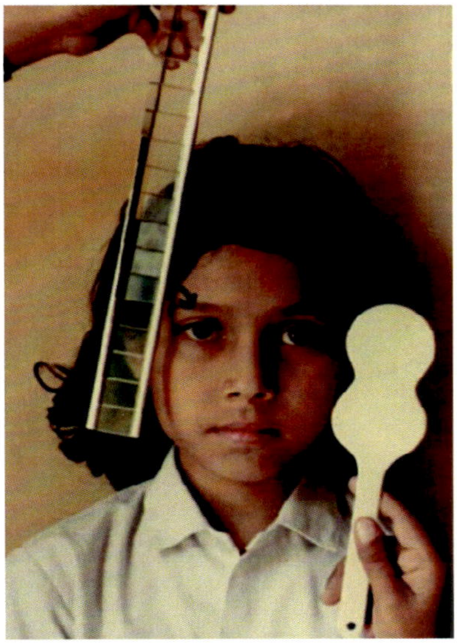

FIG. 10.10: Prism bar test

Prism Bar Reflection Test (Krimsky's Test)

This test was done to assess the deviation objectively in cases of gross amblyopia or eccentric fixation and was performed at 33 cm. This test was similar like Hirschberg's test but from a different aspect. In this test the corneal reflection in the amblyopic eye was centered by placing appropriate prisms before the fixing eye as per the prism bar cover test principle of placing prisms. The strength of the prism required gave measurement of the angle of squint.

Synoptophore

Objective angle of deviation was determined by mean of flashing method if there was good fixation and adequate vision in either eye and the patient was cooperative. Corneal reflection method was used for patients having poor fixation in squinting eye or for uncooperative child.

Flashing Method

Dissimilar pictures like a gate and a joker were chosen. The patient was asked to look at the center of the joker slide in right tube (right eye fixing). Now the light of the right eye slide was put out by means of press button and the patient's left eye was carefully observed when he was asked to look directly at the center of the gate. If the left eye moved outwards to take up fixation, it indicated esodeviation and likewise the left tube position was then adjusted or the slide in that tube was raised or lowered (in cases of vertical movements) to eliminate movement in left eye. The reading as shown on the scale that time was the objective angle of deviation fixing right eye. Placing the joker in left tube and the gate in right the test was repeated to measure the objective angle of deviation fixing left eye.

Corneal

Reflection Method: Dissimilar pictures like a cot and a joker were chosen. The tube before the fixing eye was placed at zero except in large angle of deviation where the deviation was divided between two arms of the instrument. The patient was encouraged to look directly at the picture before fixing eye. Tube before the deviating eye was then adjusted horizontally and vertically as required so that the corneal reflection in that eye coincide as accurately as possible with the same in fixing eye. Reading from the scale at this point was the objective angle of deviation measured by corneal reflection method.

Subjective Angle of Deviation

Dissimilar pictures like a gate and a joker were chosen. First the joker was kept in the right tube and the patient was asked to look directly at this. Left arm of the instrument was then moved horizontally and vertically as required so that the joker was completely into the gate. The scale reading as noted was the subjective angle of deviation fixing right eye. Placing the joker in left tube and moving the right arm of the instrument the test was repeated to measure the subjective angle of deviation fixing left eye.

By comparing subjective and objective angles of deviation, anomalous retinal correspondence was noted for its presence or absence.

The angle of deviation was measured subjectively or objectively with each eye fixing in turn in all the cardinal directions of gaze and was recorded in a table form.

Assessment of Binocular Functions (On Synoptophore)

Simultaneous macular perception (SMP) was already ascertained while measuring the subjective angle of deviation with dissimilar simultaneous perception slides.

Fusion was checked with similar slides with different controls like a tree with a boy and a tree with a girl.

After appropriate adjustment of the tubes the two pictures got superimposed and a single picture with both the controls were seen by the patient. The angle at which the fusion occurred was noted. Thereafter, fusion range was seen in abduction and adduction when the tubes were moved accordingly in coordinated manner while the patient tried to maintain the fusion of the images.

Stereopsis was noted after putting the stereoscopic slides such as those of a different color wickets and a ball while the patient was asked to tell the position of middle wicket—whether straight or inclined to any side.

The Maddox rod consists of several rods or grooves, colored red and mounted in a disk so that it refracts light rays in one direction and converts a point of light source into a red line of light when placed in front of an eye.

Method: The Maddox rod with its grooves horizontal was placed in front of one eye, while keeping the fixation of spot light (at 6 meters distance) by other eye. In exodeviation the images crossed and in esodeviation the images did not cross. The amount of deviation was measured by a prism bar till the spot light image was on the vertical line.

Vertical deviations can be ascertained and measured also in similar manner keeping the Maddox rod grooves vertical and placing base down prisms for hyperdeviation and base up prisms for hypodeviations. The whole test was repeated keeping Maddox rod in front of the other eye and the readings were recorded separately.

Maddox Wing Test

The patient was asked to look through two horizontal apertures made in the instrument holding the instrument in such a manner as required in day-to-day near working conditions. After some time he was asked to tell the number under which the two arrows, red and white, came to rest. The number under which the white arrow came to rest indicated the amount of horizontal deviation in prism diopters while that of the red arrow indicated the vertical deviation in prism diopters.

This test was applicable to small angle deviations with no suppression.

Near Point of Convergence

This was measured with the help of a RAF near point rule, the face piece of the instrument was placed on the cheek bones and the patient was instructed to look at the line marked on the card which was moved near to the eyes till the line became double or blurred. This gave the subjective measurement of the near point of convergence. While performing the test the eyes of the patient were under constant observation till either eye or both stopped converging or diverged. This gave the reading for objective near point of convergence.

Near Point of Accommodation

This was also measures with the RAF near point rule in the same way when the patient was asked to look at the letters printed on the card instead of a line. When he first noticed the letters becoming blurred was the near point of accommodation.

The near point of accommodation was measured uniocularly as well as binocularly.

Worth's Four Dot Test

The apparatus consists of a box containing four apertures of colored glasses illuminated internally — the two lateral apertures are green, the upper one red and the lower one white.

6/6 method: The patient was seated at 6 meters distance from the box wearing red green goggles, red glass being in front of right eye. If the patient had binocular single vision he would see four dots. If the patient had any manifest or latent deviation he would see five dots. The patient would see two red dots in cases of suppression of left eye and three green dots in suppression of right eye. If a patient saw four dots in presence of manifest deviation it indicated anomalous retinal correspondence. In presence of binocular single vision the color of the lower spot as seen, indicated which eye was dominant.

Bagolini's Striated Glass Test

This test was carried out by asking the patient to fixate binocularly on a spot light, after being provided with plano lenses with narrow fine striations accross one meridian. The lenses were placed with the striations perpendicular to each other. When the cross seen by the patient bisected the fixation light (at 6 meters or 33 cm) it indicated harmonious anomalous retinal correspondence in presence of a manifest squint. If only one line was seen passing through the light there was total suppression of other eye. If any line was discontinuous at the light it meant fixation point scotoma. If the light was seen double with one line passing through each, this was an indication of a manifest squint with NRC when the distance between the two spots of light was consistent with the angle of deviation; within harmonious ARC when the distance was different.

Sighting/Pointing Test

The test determined as to which eye the subject preferred in aiming or pointing at an object or in aligning two objects at different distances. The patient was asked to hold a pencil in both bands at fully stretched arm length and point it at the spot light (at 6 meters) once he has aligned the two, one eye was covered and he was asked whether the spot light and pencil were still in line or had moved out of alignment. The eye with which alignment was maintained are covering the other eye, was the dominant eye **(Fig. 10.11).**

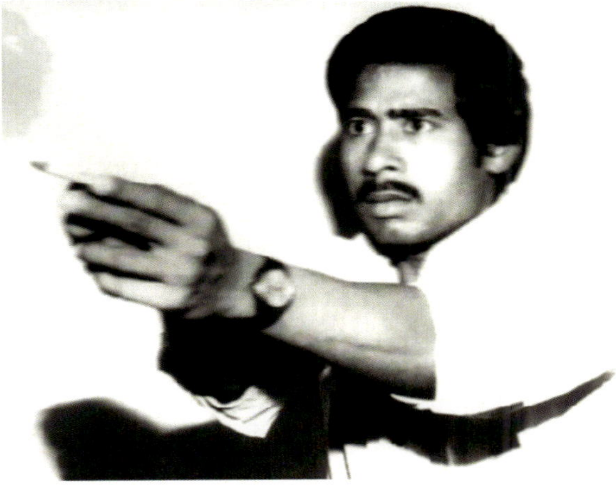

FIG. 10.11: Sighting (fixation test)

After Image Test on Synoptophore *(Fig. 10.12)*

The right eye slide had horizontal line with central red spot and the left had vertical line with central red spot. Each eye in turn was stimulated for about 20 seconds and during this period the corneal reflections were monitored to ensure central fixation. After stimulating each eye in turn, the automatic binocular flashing device was switched on.

The patient observed one of the following:

i. A patient with NRC saw a symmetrical cross.
ii. In patient with ARC there was a horizontal (or rarely vertical) shift.

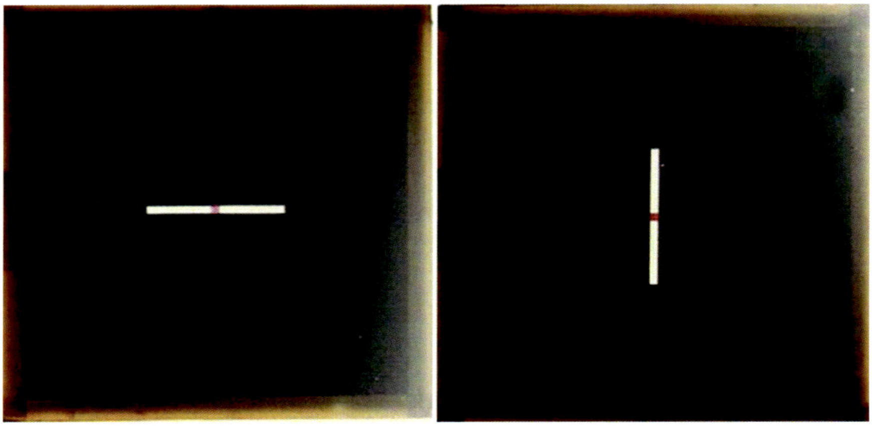

FIG. 10.12: After image test of synaptophore

iii. Some patients, however, suppressed too strongly to appreciate one of the after images.

Refraction and Fundus Examination

Retinoscopy was carried out with the help of streak retinoscope or plane mirror retinoscope under the effect of full mydriasis and cycloplegia in each eye. Atropine 1% ointment twice daily for three days was used in young children; in older children and young adults 1% cyclopentolate eyedrops or homatropine eyedrops was used for mydriasis and cycloplegia. Postmydriatic test was done days after when the effect of the mydriatic had passed off.

Under the effect of mydriasis, fundus examination was carried out in each eye with direct ophthalmoscope to note the condition of the media, optic disk, blood vessels, macular region, fovea and general periphery of the central fundus. A careful search was made for any abnormality or any ocular sign of systemic diseases like meningitis, benign intracranial hypertension, diabetes, etc.

Fixation was checked also in each eye with the pupil dilated (it can be done in undilated pupil also) with the help of Heine's direct ophthalmoscope having a special device (a star and concentric rings) incorporated in it for examination of fixation, which can be removed when desired. The target was presented first to the normal eye(or to the eye with better visual acuity) so that the patient could recognize the target and his cooperation was assessed. Other eye being occluded the patient was asked to see the target star. The location of it in respect with the foveal reflex as seen by the examiner was noted. The target was moved and refixation checked. Confirmation of accuracy of fixation was also obtained by asking the patient to fixate on different parts of the target. Fixation as observed was recorded as foveal, unsteady foveal, erratic or unsteady parafoveal, parafoveal, paramacular, centrocecal, paracecal, divergent and nonfixation. Fixation was also recorded as steady or unsteady. The whole method was repeated for the other eye also.

Eccentric Viewing vs Eccentric Fixation

1. Eccentric viewing is an intermediate stage between central and eccentric fixation reflex remain oriented towards the fovea, although foveal function is reduced. In eccentric fixation the fixation reflex becomes adjusted to nonfoveal (Paramacular) retinal elements. Eccentric viewing is frequently present in macular retinopathy.

We can differentiate between eccentric fixation and eccentric viewing by visuoscope.

Method: The sound eye is occluded. The examiner projects the visuoscope asterisk (Star) into (onto) the retinal periphery of the patient. We ask the patient to look directly at the asterisk. Firstly there will be an eye movement so that the image of the fixation target can form on fovea but the image will be very dim because foveal function of the patient is reduced (Scotoma, organic lesion). Secondly, the eye will move (again?) so that now the image from fovea can move to peripheral retinal element, where visual acuity may be better than in the fovea. Eccentric viewing is present.

2. The first eye movement, displaces the asterisk directly to the fovea. The fixation reflex has adopted itself to peripheral nasal retinal elements. Eccentric fixation is present.

CONCOMITANT SQUINT METHOD OF EXAMINATION

Qualitative Diagnosis of Strabismus

1. Cover test for detection of heterotrophia
2. Indirect cover test
3. Cover uncover test for detection of heterophoria.

Quantitative Diagnosis of Strabismus

1. Hischberg test
2. Prism reflex test of Krimsky

3. Prism cover test
4. Maddox rod test for heterophoria
5. Prism dissociation test
6. Maddox double prism test for cyclodeviation
7. Maddox double rod test for cyclodeviation
8. Diplopia test for measurement of ocular deviation.

TREATMENT

The main aim of treatment is to:

1. Attain normality of appearance
2. To restore binocular single vision in all circumstances.

There are four methods by which a patient can be treated.

Glasses

i. Glasses improve visual acuity
ii. Lessens or overcome angle of deviation.

Treatment of Amblyopia

It will be discussed in subsequent chapter.

Orthoptic Treatment

The aim is to restore or development of normal function. A number of patients who has a weak binocular vision or suppression of the more ametropic eye an effort was make to build binocular vision with orthoptic exercises as follows:

Antisuppression Exercises

On cherioscope and chasing and flashing exercises on major amblyoscope were with the use of simultaneous macular perception slides. It was given in those cases who has complete or partial suppression of more ametropic eye with a view to provide stimulus to the suppressed eye. The exercises were given 10 to 15 minutes daily.

Fusion Exercises

Fusion exercises on major amblyoscope: Fusion exercises were given on the major amblyoscope with the fusion slides fusion range could be increased by gradually converging both the tube is of major amblyoscope till the fusion breaks.

Exercises were give daily or on alternate days for 10 to 15 minutes depending on the tolerance and convenience of the patient.

Fusion exercises on diploscope: It is based on physiological diplopia and requires simultaneous use of the eyes.

Home exercises: Home exercises comprising of convergence to near point, (Pencil to nose exercise) and reorganization of physiological diplopia for near and distance were explained to the patient. Patients were instructed to do the exercises almost two to three times daily for 10 to 15 minutes.

Operation

Surgery is required for residual angle of squint which is not corrected by glasses in case of accommodative squint. Give preorthoptic exercise in divergent squint to improve the binocular function but it should not be persisted for long time otherwise convergence spasm will develop, and then, surgery is advocated. The aim of operation is to restore visual axes to parallelism in all direction of gaze. In neglected cases where surgery is carried on for cosmetic reason, one should leave a few degrees of convergence. Since in the passage of time subsequent divergence may occur.

A. Various weaking operation or extrinsic ocular muscles are:
   1. Recession
   2. Marginal myotomy.

B. Lengthening operation on extrinsic ocular muscles are:
   1. Simple tenotomy
   2. Resection.

AMOUNT OF OPERATION

Following empirical rules are useful in chalking out a preoperative plan.

1. The larger the deviation, the greater will be the effect of surgery.
2. Long-standing deviation (with secondary changes) will require more surgery then recent deviation.
3. More effect is produced per mm of recession or resection in a child or in patient with small eyes than in an adult or patient with larger eyes.
4. Recession is more effective than resection in reducing deviations.

5. If fusion is present a cure with fusion may be expected, a slight over-correction help obtain the result but if no fusion potential is present, a slight under correction visual produce a stable small angle residual deviation.
6. The presence of amblyopia makes the result of surgery unpredictable and all such patient should be warned of the possibility of a second operation.
7. Esodeviation or exodeviation greater than 50 Δ in a patient with very poor vision in one eye should be treated with a supramaximal recession surgery one eye to avoid surgery on better eye.
8. Three muscle surgery for esotropia or exotropia may be required for deviation greater than 50 Δ but less than 60°.
9. 4 muscle surgery for deviation more than 60°.

Anterior Segment Ischemia

Anterior segment of eye is supplied by 7 anterior ciliary and 2 postciliary arteries when we do disinsection of the recti, we divide there anterior ciliary arteries and loss of blood to the three muscles (below the age of 26 years) and more than 2 muscles in older patient produces some degree of anterior segment ischemia.

Symptoms and Sign of Anterior Segment Ischemia

Pain, blurring of vision, edema of lid, conjunctiva and cornea, deep anterior chamber with heavy flare, iris atrophy, iris angiography shows poor arterial filling.
Treatment: Atropine, topical and systemic steroids.

Faden Operation or Postfixation Suture

It is the weakening procedure on the contralateral synergist muscle of a paralytical lateral rectus. When the muscle is recessed the distance between muscle's origin and insertion is decreased and muscle becomes slack but in Faden operation the muscle is attached to globe although we pass strong posterior fixation suture in the muscle belly so there is no slackness of muscle. Postfixation suture must be strong we can use 3-0 supramid. There are two methods of carrying out Faden's operation—strong permanent sutures are applied 13mm behind its undetached insertion (The appropriate distance of applying posterior fixation suture in case of medial rectus muscle is 13 mm, it is 17 mm in the case of lateral rectus).

First we recess the muscle by 3 mm and then we pass the posterior fixation suture 13 mm behind the detached insertion.

In Faden operation the effect of recession is increased because all muscle slackness is taken up by the short length of muscle between the suture and its point of origin.

This procedure is used on rectus. In DVD (dissociated vertical divergence) we can use this method to reduce elevation of superior. Rectus by this operation we can increase the effect of recession operation we can perform this operation in infantile esotropia and nystagmus blockage syndrome.

Adjustable Sutures

Adjustable sutures are useful where it is difficult to predict the result of conventional recession therapy, e.g. in intermittent.

1. Divergence excess type of exotropia
2. Vertical muscle palsy
3. Cosmetic operation in older patients where there is risk of postoperative diplopia
4. Consecutive exotropia.

The recessed muscle must be sutured in such a way so that postoperatively the muscle tendon can be drawn forward or backward at the time of adjustment (The conjunctival incision has to be left open so that the muscle sutures are easily accessible). This operation is unsuitable in children below 15 years.

ACCOMMODATIONAL SQUINT

Before dealing with accommodational squint proper, it is certain to understand the mechanism of accommodation and convergence as well as their mutual relationship.

Physiology

The association between accommodation and convergence such that when each eye undergoes the required amount of accommodation in order see a near object. Hence a satisfactory accommodation–convergence synkinesis results within the occipital cortex and this is an inborn, unconditioned reflex. Accommodation measurement is expressed in diopters and convergence in meter angle. In order to see clearly an object placed at 1 meter the eye requires one diopter of accommodation as well as 1 meter while of convergence in each eye. Convergence sometimes is also depressed in terms of prism diopters, 1 meter angle being equivalent to three prism diopters.

Under normal conditions, the convergence is influenced not only by accommodation but also by (i) tone of extrinsic ocular muscles, (ii) proximity of the object and (iii) fusional impulses. Therefore the total convergence is composed of the following components.

Accommodative Convergence

It is that part of convergence which is brought about in response to the act of accommodation.

Proximal Convergence

This reflex is stimulated by the sense of nearness of the object and seems to be independent of accommodation.

Tonic Convergence

It is that convergence which determine position of the visual axis in relation to each other when eyes are in primary position, fixing a distant object. It depends on the light that strikes the retina and impulses that arise in the labyrinths, neck and trunk muscles.

Fusional Convergence

As a result of this reflex the eyes are directed to objects of attention and interest and are maintained in such a position relative to each other so that the images of object of fixation fall on the fovea of each eye simultaneously this reflex exerts a very important influence upon accommodative convergence. For relationship example, in cases of superable, corrected hypermetropia a greater amount of accommodation is called for, to see a near object clearly. This act of accommodation could in itself simulate an equal amount of accommodative convergence which being excessive would produce a convergent squint. This however, does not happen in all cases of uncorrected hypermetropia because parallelism in these cases is thought to be maintained by fusional convergence which exerts an influence on accommodative convergence to nullify the excess of convergence stimulated by excessive accommodation. Similarly, in case of uncorrected myopia a reduced amount of accommodation would be needed for fixing a near object thereby stimulating a lesser amount of convergence. In this case, the fusional convergence comments the deficit in accommodative convergence and a single binocular vision is maintained. That part of fusional convergence which adjusts a deficit of convergence is called positive relative fusional convergence and that which adjusts the excess of convergence is called negative relative fusional convergence. The fusional convergence is believed to be mediated through a center in the frontal cortex. If the power to inhibit convergence by fusional reserve (i.e. negative relative fusional convergence) exceeds the excessive convergence stimulated by hypermetropia, a squint does not develop. On the other hand, in a case of hypermetropia where accommodative convergence exceeds the inhibitory power, manifest convergent squint results.

Accommodative Convergence/Accommodation (AC/A) Ratio

The amount of accommodative convergence measured in prism diopters induced by each diopter of accommodation is called the AC/A ratio. The average value is 3:1 to 5:1 which is usually expressed as 3 to 5 because convergence measured is related to one diopter of accommodation.

Accommodating Squint

Accommodative convergent squint is that squint in which convergent deviation of the eyes varies according to the amount of accommodation exerted. Due to late development of the ciliary muscle, and child does not start taking interest in near objects before the age of two years, squint rarely occurs before the age of 2-2 years although sometimes it starts at the age of one year.

Classification

Causes in which binocular single vision is present in certain circumstances.

Fully Accommodative Type

Those who when wearing correct glasses enjoy binocular visual acuity but who when not wearing glasses who a convergent deviation or a reduction of their binocular visual acuity if they control the tendency to deviate.

Convergence—Excess Type

Binocular single vision with full binocular visual acuity is present for distance but there is usually a manifest deviation for near vision even with glasses. This type falls broadly speaking into two groups.

Group A: In this group the defect appears to be related to hypermetropia. In these cases some factor is superadded causing overconvergence in near vision such a factor may be (a) proximal convergence reflex, (b) defect in the subjective appreciation of the distance of an object from the observer, (c) a congenital defect in the action of extrinsic ocular muscle.

Group B: In this group – (a) the degree of hyper is lower or there may be no refractive error, (b) additional plus lens do not reduce the manifest deviation for near vision and may sometimes cause it to increase, (c) There is frequently a vertical defect in addition to manifest convergence in near vision, (d) The AC/A ratio is markedly higher than normal, (e) There is marked inability to exercise negative relative personal convergence.

Divergence–Insufficiency Type

There is a manifest convergent squint for distance of esophoria for near. It is sometime associated with congenital tropia and following miotic therapy.

Cases in Which Binocular Single Vision is Absent

Partially Accommodative Type

Visual axis are convergent in all circumstances but deviation increase where accommodation is exerted and when hypermetropia correction is removed. This group may be further subdivided:

i. Those patients with normal binocular function
ii. Those patients without binocular function
iii. Those who have very weak or anomalous binocular function.

Clinical Investigations

History

When taking the history of squint from the parent it is important to make sure that the two eyes are not looking in the one direction because the word 'squinting' is sometimes used to imply 'screwing up of the eyelids'. One should attempt to discover (a) precisely what the parent or other observer has noticed miss with the child's eyes and at what age this anomaly was first noticed, (b) whatever eye is going in or out, (c) whether the squint unilateral or bilateral or each eye, (d) whether the squint intermittent or constant, (e) whether squint is increasing, decreasing or stationary, (f) whether squint increases or decreases in various times of day, and (g) from how long he is using the glasses. Whether angle of squint increases with glasses or it remains the same.

The extent to which various tests need to be carried out tend soon the characteristics of the condition, age and cooperation of the patient and the duration of the squint allowing tests would cover the examination required in most of the cases.

Refraction and Visual Acuity

Acuity should be tested with and without glasses both for near and distance.

Refraction: The refractive state of the eye should be carefully determined under full cycloplegia so as to uncover total hypermetropia.

Orthoptics Investigations

While doing this test care should be taken to see that accommodation is fully excreted. For this purpose, a small letter for the test type may be used for distance and small letters or picture on the near fixation bar.

Cover Test

Ocular movements: These should be tested with care so as to detect any 'A' or 'V' phenomenon or any vertical anomaly.

Examination with Major Amblyoscope

It is important in increasing the state of binocular function. The measurement of the angle of deviation should be undertaken with and without glasses.

Measurement of Near Point of Accommodation

There are several methods which can be both uniocular and binocular.

Estimation of the AC/A Ratio

There are several methods which can be employed to measure the AC/A ratio.

Estimation of Negative and Positive Fusional Convergence

As already stated every effort of accommodation is accompanied by accommodative convergence. If this accommodative convergence is excessive it is inhibited by negative relative fusional convergence of fusional convergence should be made by the following method test is performed with the patients wearing correcting glasses throughout the test.

i. The patient is asked to read the smallest possible line of Snellen chart placed at 6 meter distance. The fact that he is fixing binocularly can be verified by cover test.
ii. Minus spherical lens are inserted before the eyes starting with 0.5D and then increasing the strength in stages by -0.5D convergent squint appears. The value of greatest minus lens which dermits a clear single binocular vision is recorded.
iii. The test is repeated with convex lens similarly and the limit of clear vision recorded.
iv. The whole test is repeated at 33.3 cm using a small satisfactory result for this test with the ability to maintain clear binocular single vision up to the value of –4.0D for distance and –5.0D sph. For near vision, this test has been described as a result for relative accommodation, it being assured that accommodation can be altered when lens are introduced without any need to inhibit the accompanying change in convergence. This appears most unlikely and it is suggested that the term "relative accommodation" is discontinued.

Treatment

Although individual cases merit individualized treatment, a general line of treatment may be described as follows:

Correction of Refraction Error

It should be done at the earliest possible age so that further development of the habit of suppression, when accommodation is exerted is prevented. The refraction should be done under complete cycloplegia to correct full hypermetropia. Over correction of hypermetropia is not desirable regular procedure because it tends insufficiency in later life. Over correction has its balance especially in children too young for subjective testing provided the over correction secures parallelism of visual axis but it should never be continued for a prolonged period, any decrease in distant visual acuity on account of this procedure should be explained to the parents.

Occlusion

Due to late onset of squint and often being intermittent in character it is unusual to find a marked degree of amblyopia in fully accommodative squint. The inhibition of the fovea in early stage of squint may lead to amblyopia to avoid confusion. The correct spectacle should be worn constantly and child should be examined at frequent intervals during initial stage of occlusion. When partial occlusion is employed the parent and teacher must try to ensure that the child does not give up the glasses otherwise the condition is aggravated by excessive use of accommodation. Occlusion may cause than angle of squint to increase.

Orthoptic Treatment

Orthoptic treatment for those cases in which binocular single vision is present.

Indications: This treatment is indicated when (i) the clinical shows a manifest deviation when glasses are removed, (ii) he does not appreciate diplopia, (iii) he is unable to straighten his eyes for near fixation.

The treatment may be divided into four stages:

1. To overcome suppression, particularly at the convergent angle of deviation.
2. To teach the patient relaxation of accommodation and convergence.
3. To teach the patient negative relative fusional convergence and to improve binocular visual acuity.
4. To ensure that the patient has good binocular convergence.

Overcoming Suppression

In giving treatment on the major amblyoscope in order to overcome suppression when accommodation takes place, the patient should be made to exert 3 diopters of accommodation either by the insertion of -2D spherical lens in the lens holders of the major amblyoscope, in which case he should wear his glasses, or by using lens which are equal to the patients correction with -3D sphere added. Antisuppression exercises such as chasing in and out should be given the use of simultaneous perception slides, with foveal sized fixation picture helps to ensure that full accommodation is exerted.

The following exercises may be practiced both in the clinic or at home.

i. ***Optometric exercises***: Wearing red and green glasses the patient is instructed to practice making a spot light appear alternately red and green. If possible, this exercise should being carried out thought the correcting lens being worn. At first he may need help by means of rapid alternating covering of the eyes.

ii. ***Diplopia***: Patients who are sufficiently cooperative should be brought to recognize diplopia when squinting and those who can attain binocular single vision may practice recognizing physical diplopia.

The cheiroscope and the pigeon cantonnet stereoscope to valuable for overcoming suppression.

Teaching Relaxation of Accommodation

At this stage of treatment diplopia should be appropriated so that patient can instruct how to join the double images to one. However should include that child should practice maintaining single image. This is an indication to him that his eyes have become straight.

Using a major amblyoscope, the patient should be thought to relax accommodation while the angle of the tubes is used to zero or as near zero as possible. The correction for the patient's hypermetropia should be reduced by the use of appropriate/lenses inserted into lens holder. Fusion or stereoscopic picture should be used for exercise; the image will become increasingly blurred as the visual axes approach parallelism.

When amblyopia has been corrected suppression, the patient has been taught to control/upon his power of negative relative fusional convergence. If this is found to be adequate, treatment/may be discontinued apart from wearing the glass. Patient should report for regular follow up examinations. The strength of the glasses should be reduced when negative relative fusion convergence seems able to control the additional accommodative convergence. If negative relative fusional convergence is found to be deficient or patient is further/treatment may be undertaken to increase the power of inhibiting accommodative convergence and increasing negative relative fusional convergence.

Teaching Negative Relative Fusional, Convergence and Improving Binocular Visual Acuity

There are a variety of instruments which may be used in carrying out these exercises, such instruments include the major amblyoscope bar Reader, Holmes and Asher law stereoscopes, remiseparator and stereorgrance cards held in the hand.

With a major amblyoscope exercises may be given during a gradual reduction of the patient's hypermetropic correction the –1.D sphere are placed in the lens holders of the instruments during simple fusion slides he is to describe the picture as accurately as he can taking care that it does not become double and that suppression does not occur. When he does this, 2.D later – 3D sphere should be substituted and more detailed slides should be used in place of simpler one. Fusion should be maintained as near to zero as possible and adduction exercises should then be practiced while patient is asked to maintain a single clear vision.

Teaching Good Binocular Convergence

Simple convergence exercises should be taught and may be practised at home, care being taken to ensure that accurate convergence take place without suppression of either eye. The patient should be encouraged to be aware of physiological diplopia when convergence fails.

Binocular convergence may also be improved by use of sterograme/ cards held in hand and by use of a prism bar and also by convergence exercises using the major amblyoscope.

Miotic Therapy

Miotics are drugs which stimulate accommodation peripherally by contraction of ciliary muscle and also constrict the pupil. By virtue of pupil contriction, clearity of vision is improved and by both these peripheral actions there is a abduction in subjective effort of accommodation in order to see clearly. A reduction in the subjective effort of accommodation less accommodation convergence, the result being that clear vision is achieved without the accurance of a manifact convergent deviation. Miotics are said to be useful for a child also young for orthoptic treatment. They are also helpful postoperatively if a convergent deviation still occurs on accommodation.

Prerequisite

i. Equal visual acuity in either eye
ii. Absence of suppression
iii. Presence of fusion with a good range fusion
iv. Binocular single vision for distance (with glasses if worn)
v. Binocular single vision for near when using the miotics.

The miotics most commonly used are:

i. Pilocarpine 1%
ii. DFP (di-isopropyl fluorophosphonate) .005%, 01%
iii. PI (Phospholine iodide) 0.06%, 0.125% or 0.25% 0.25%.

iv. Pilocarpine is instilled three times daily being later reduced as the binocular visual acuity improves.

Disadvantage

Its action wars off within a few hour. This provides a practical difficulty with children who are at the school all day.

DFP needs only one instillation every 24 hrs. The drops are susceptible to absorption of moisture so parents should be warned to keep the bottle tightly stoppered.

Phospholine iodide is usually instilled once each twenty hour and given at night. At first a solution of 0.25% or 0.125% may be used but subsequently this may be reduced to 0.06%.

It is important that miotic therapy should be continued with orthoptic exercises, including home exercises. Throughout the treatment there should be regular and careful supervision of the patient in the orthoptic department. The patient should be examined to see if there is any appearance of yet in the pigment layers of iris. In some cases there have occurred where the drug has been given over a prolonged period, but this is lees likely to occur when the strength of drops does not exceed 0.25%.

Surgical Treatment

In some case optical and orthoptic treatment to eliminate manifest squint near fixation, surgical treatment in indicated to achieve binocular single vision for all distances on fixation. It is important to uncover the full amount of variation with and without glasses by making the patient exert all accommodation while determining the angle of squint both for near and distance.

Although on theoretical grounds a bilateral recession of redial recti might be considered as the operation of choices, recess the medial rectus and resect the ipsilateral medial rectus thus leaving the opposite eye for further surgery undertaken in cases of convergence excess type of binocular function is good.

If the child is old enough the operation should both loaded and followed by appropriate orthoptic exercise in order to achieve maximum binocular function. In the case of young child surgery may be postponed if the deviation is not frequent and there is no danger of disturbance in the binocular function.

Criteria for Cure

The patient should have comfortable binocular vision with and without glasses for near and distance. If the hypermetropia exceeds + 3D binocular single vision should be maintained when correction reduced by 3 diopters. Binocular visual acuity with classes should be equal to visual acutiy of each eye or of the weaker eye if it is so.

The patient should be able to bar read N5 with glasses and also where -3D is added to them.

Binocular convergence be 8 cm and should be well-maintained.

Just to Summary the Accommodation Squint

Esotropia (Convergent squint)

i. Accommodational esotropia
ii. Nonaccommodational esotropia.

Accommodational ESO is associated with the without (N) accommodation. A normal person or one with normal refractive error in order to see a nearly object, he has to make his lens convex. It is done by contraction of ciliary muscles.

Accommodative Squint

Relaxation of suspensory ligament. Normally, the lens is kept flattened by suspensory ligaments.

During accommodation there is contraction of ciliary muscle and relaxation of suspensory ligament—Lens becomes convex in hypermetropia which is undercorrected or uncorrected person requires more accommodation (over accommodation) so requires over convergence.

Another type of accommodative esotropia.

- Not associated with any refractive error. This is because of neuromuscular abnormality.
- Age–2-3 years.
- Family history of squint is present.
- To start with it is intermittent in nature but later it becomes constant. It is more for near than for distance.
- Cover test in accommodative squint — should use a fixation bar with a picture over it instead of a torch. This compel the child to accommodate in order to see properly.

Treatment of Accommodative Eso

- Refraction under full cycloplegia 1% atropine drop BD × 3 days.
- Give full correction.
- One deviation is corrected the no. of glasses paper step by step when deviation is absent for distance and present for near bifocal lenses with increased number for near or give miotic treatment.

– Pilocarpine BD

Or Phosphoeria iodido

Or DFP (rarely).

Action of Mioties

Peripheral stimulation of accommodation and constriction of pupil so that child sees clearly, central accommodation does not come into play.

Indication of Miotic Theory

i. Small or no refractive error
ii. Equal and good visual acuity
iii. When AC/A ratio is increased.

Treatment by surgery:

i. For nonaccommodation part of squint.
ii. If amblyopia is present—treatment improves the visual acuity.
iii. Visual acuity poor. Treatment of amblyopia.
iv. Improve BF by orthoptic treatment
v. Nonaccommodational squint—surgery is advocated.

EXODEVIATION

Introduction

Generally speaking divergent squint develops due to breakdown of binocular reflexes before they are become adequately strong. As comparison to convergent squint, divergent squint is less common, the ratio being 1:4. The divergent squint is more common in females. It tends to increase with age. It may pass through latent, or intermittent phase and it may be absent in the morning and tends to increase with fatigue towards the end of the day. Usually, there is no refractive error. Amblyopia and abnormal retinal correspondence are rare in

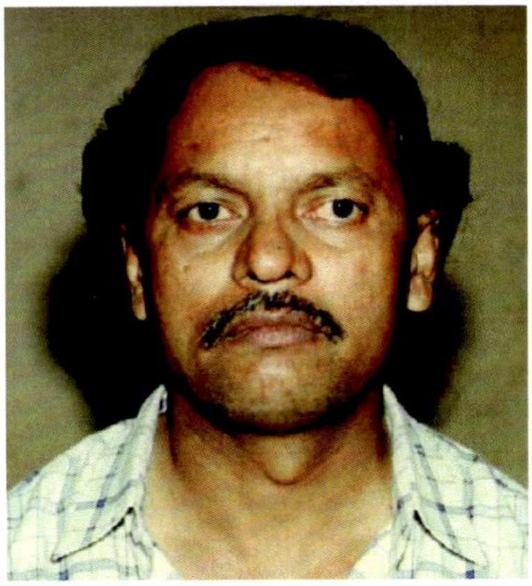

FIG. 10.13: Divergent squint

exodeviation. To start with there may be diplopia but later on suppression develops.

Exodeviation can be defined as divergent alignment of the visual axes **(Fig. 10.13).** It may be exophoria intermittent exotropia or constant exotropia. In exophoria, the deviation is held latent by the fusional and accommodative convergence reflexes. Exodeviation is developed either due to excessive tonic divergent or due to deficient tonic convergence.

Classification

Exodeviation can be classified into following patterns (Duane's classification):

1. *Divergence excess pattern*: The exodeviation is at least 15Δ larger at distance than at near fixation.
2. *Basic exodeviation*: The distance deviation is approximately equal to the near deviation.
3. *Convergence insufficiency pattern*: The near deviation is at least 15Δ greater than the distance deviation.
4. *Simulated divergence excess pattern*: The prism bar and cover test will show an exodeviation which is significantly larger at distance than at near fixation. The static deviation at near fixation is obscured by dynamic factors like persistent convergence innervation, and special tests are required to reveal the deviation at near fixation which will then often equal or even exceed that at distant fixation. This can be also of two types pseudodivergence excess Type I and pseudodivergence excess Type II.

Exodeviation can also be of following types:

1. Primary exodeviation
2. Secondary exodeviation—due to loss of vision in one eye.
3. Consecutive exodeviation—due to over correction of convergent squint.

Investigation

History

Investigations start with the history. In exodeviation, certain points to be noted during taking history:

1. Mode of deviation—Outward deviation suggests exodeviation.
2. Age of onset—Age of onset of the majority of the cases of exodeviation is usually late. That is why retraining is better in case of exodeviations
3. Mode of onset—Exodeviations begin as an exophoria which may deteriorate into intermittent and constant exotropia, as suppression occurs.
4. Progression of deviation—The deviation increases in condition of Fatigue or ill-health. Divergence excess type of deviation tends to remain more or less static, whereas with simulated divergence excess type the near deviation tends to increase. In convergence weakness pattern, there is a tendency for the deviation to increase.
5. Ocular symptom—In exophoria and intermittent exotropia patient may complaint of following symptoms:
   - Blurred vision
   - Difficulty in focusing
   - Difficulties with prolonged period of near work, headache
   - Eyeache
   - Diplopia
   - Photophobia
   - Micropsia.
6. *History of using spectacles or prisms*: Exodeviation may occur in acquired myopia, unilateral anisometropic myopia or in myopic astigmatism. So there may be history of using spectacles for those refractive errors. There may also be history of using base—in prisms in case of exodeviation.
7. *Family history*: In exodeviation, there is frequently a family history of squint.

Visual Acuity

Visual acuity is tested both uniocularly and binocularly with or without glasses. It is tested both for distance and near.

In primary exodeviation, amblyopia is the exception rather than rule, but if the deviation is constant and unilateral, there may be some defect of visual acuity or suppression in the squinting eye.

In intermittent exodeviation, there may be impaired binocular visual acuity due to over exercise of convergence and consequently accommodation in order to achieve control of the deviation.

In presbyopia exophoria or intermittent exodeviation may occur.

Refraction

In exodeviation some refraction errors may be detected—like acquired myopia, unilateral anisometropic myopia or myopic astigmatism.

Exophoria my be found with

a. Bilateral acquired myopia, due to reduction in the demand for accommodative efforts.
b. Presbyopia, as the near point recedes and the bond between accommodation and convergence is weakened.

External, Examination

To rule our pseudoexodeviation external ovular examination is carried out. Pseudoexodeviation may be produced by:

1. A large positive angle alpha
2. Wide interpupillary distance
3. Exophthalmos
4. A wide palpebral fissure.

Head Posture

Chin elevation – in some cases of exodeviation chin is slightly elevated in order to favor a more convergent position of the eyes associated with depression.

Cover Test (Fig. 10.14)

In exodeviation, cover test is performed at 1/3 meter, 6 meters and at far distance, beyond 6 meters.

Depending on the type of exodeviation the cover test may give the following informations:

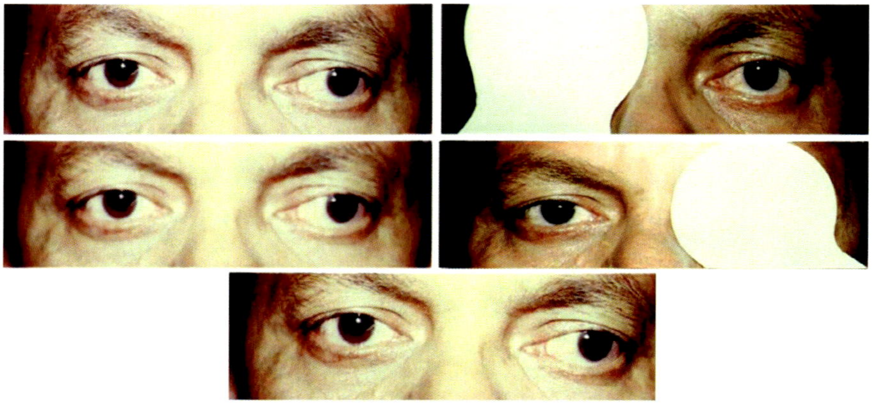

FIG. 10.14: Cover test in a case of left divergent squint

1. At 1/3 meter, the cover test may show manifest divergence or latent divergence with a varying rate of recovery to binocular single vision or without any spontaneous recovery.
2. At 6 meters, the cover test may show manifest divergence or latent divergence with a varying rate of recovery to binocular single vision or without any spontaneous recovery.
3. At far distance beyond 6 meters, the deviation may be manifest or latent. Testing in this position is important when examining a case of intermittent exodeviation of the divergence excess pattern in which the deviation is well-controlled for fixation at 6 meters distance.
4. Cover test in straight up-gaze and straight down–gaze may elicit the presence of 'A' or 'V' phenomenon.

Ocular Movements (Fig. 10.15)

In primary exodeviation, there is obvious abnormally of ocular movements. Slight palsy (paresis) of the medial rectus may be underlying cause of exophoria.

Convergence Test

In most cases of pure intermittent exodeviation, convergence is normal and well-maintained, except in the case of older patients who may develop an associated weakness of convergence.

Prism Bar and Cover Test

This test performed at 1/3 meter, at 6 meters and at far distance beyond 6 meters.

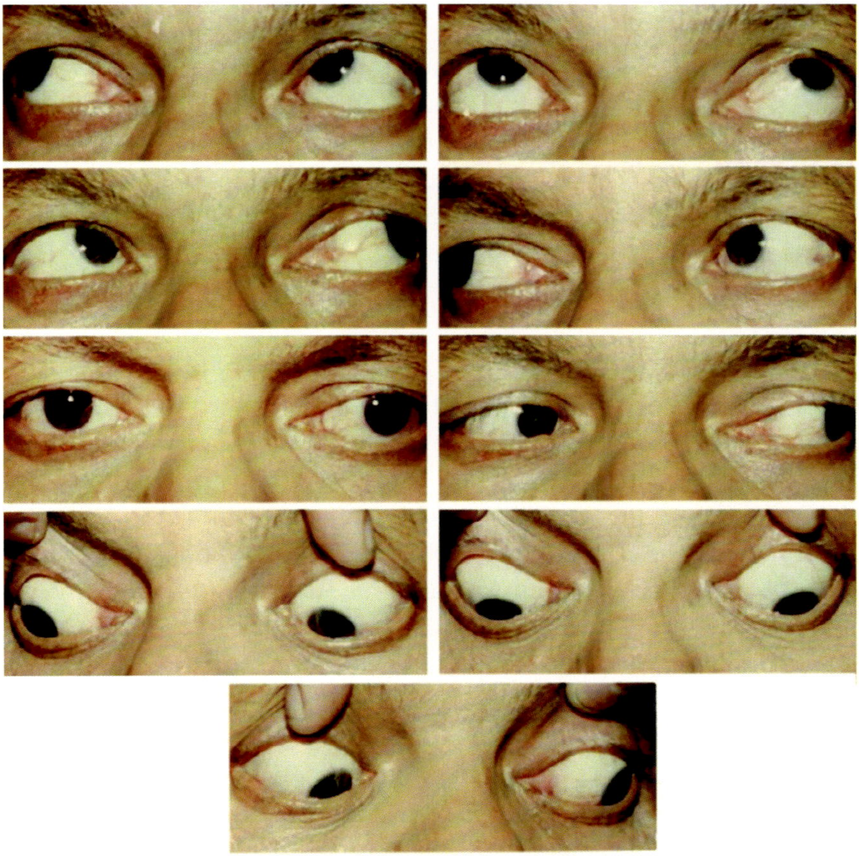

FIG. 10.15: Version in a case of left divergent squint

This test is of particular importance in the investigation of primary exodeviation because the maximum angle of deviation is more easily revealed as it does not induce unnecessary accommodation. The angle of deviation for near and distance fixation can be accurately compared. However, large deviation cannot measured by this test because of aberration produced by high prismatic power.

Maddox Wing Test

This test is done for near fixation. As accommodation is required in order to see the number clearly, the maximum angle of deviation of near fixation is not always revealed by this test. However, if the reading is compared with that of the PBCT at 1/3 meter, useful information is gained as to the amount of divergent deviation, which can be controlled. If suppression is marked, it is not possible to perform this test.

Maddox Rod Test

This is done for distance fixation (at 6 meters distance). This test is also not possible to perform in the presence of suppression.

If the deviation elicited by Maddox wing test is more than that of Maddox rod test then it indicated convergence weakness pattern of exodeviation. If the deviation elicited by Maddox rod test is more than that of Maddox wing test then it indicated divergence excess pattern of exodeviation.

Synoptophore Examination

Suppression occurs at the divergent angle. To estimate binocular function an attempt should be made in the controlled position as well as at the maximum divergent position:

a. With the deviation controlled—Good binocular function with normal retinal correspondence is usually present. Various devices may be necessary in order to stimulate accommodation and thereby maintain the controlled position. Such methods include the use of –3.0D sph, lenses before each eye, slides of exercise of convergence to a small test object.
b. At the maximum angle of divergence:
   Estimation on the synoptophore may reveal one of the following responses:
   i. Simultaneous macular perception with normal retinal correspondence. If suppression is dense, this may only be demonstrational with kinetic stimulation.
   ii. Lack of retinal correspondence due to gross suppression. The lion (fixation slide) may be seen to the right or left of the cage but disappears as the patient tries to superimpose them.
   iii. Retinal congruity—The patient is quite unable to related the two images. The lion is never seen to approach the cage.

The maximum angle deviation may be difficult to measure if the deviation is well-controlled. Alternate flashing or occlusion of one eye may help to elicit the true angle. The use of large simple slides also may help to elicit the angle.

Diplopia Test

In exodeviation, crossed diplopia or suppression of one eye may be elicited.

Special Tests for Exodeviation

In exodeviation, two special tests are carried out:

1. Occlusion test
2. +3.0D sph, lens test.

Occlusion Test

This test is done to differentiate between true and simulated divergence excess pattern. By occlusion, the fusional, the fusional stimuli is removed. After measuring the deviation with prism bar cover test at near and distant fixation, one eye in covered for 30 to 45 mins and the deviation is increased after occlusion for 30 to 45 mins. In true divergence excessive near deviation is not influenced by occlusion.

+3.0D Spherical Lens Test

+3.0D spherical lenses suspend accommodation and thus suspend accommodative convergence. In exodeviation with low AC/A ratio, the angle of deviation will increase slightly when measured through +3.0D spherical lenses. On the other hand, exodeviation with a high AC/A ratio, if the deviation is measured through +3.0D sph lenses, it will increase substantially at near fixation.

Management of Exodeviation

Optical Treatment

Refraction should be performed under cycloplegia and the correct glasses prescribed if indicated. If myopia, unilateral or bilateral, is present, its important. Small degrees of hypermetropia or hypermetropic astigmation are best left uncorrected.

Concave lens: Over-correcting concave lenses can be used to stimulate convergence by inducing accommodation thus aiding control of exodeviation concave lenses ranging in alternative from 2 to 4 D are added to the patient's refractive errors. The main value of concave lenses is to defer the surgical procedure.

Prism: Base in prism can be used to compensate the deviation in children to allow the continued binocular single vision. Prism has got no curative value. It only allows postponement of surgery.

Tinted glass: It is recognized that bright light is a dissociating factor. By reducing of light entering the eye, tinted glasses can improve the patient's control over exodeviation.

Surgical Treatment

Operation is usually necessary if a complete cure is to be obtained.

Aim of surgery: The aim of surgery is either to correct deviation or to over correct it slightly, leaving the patient with slight convergence with uncrossed diplopia. This small exodeviation usually disappears during the immediate postoperative period and the final results may be more satisfactory.

Suitable age for surgery: In extreme youth, it is rarely necessary to undertake operation so long as the deviation remains intermittent. In the case of a young child, it is better to wait until the age of four or five or even later, when cooperation for examination and treatment is more reliable.

Choice of Surgical Procedure

i. In case of true divergence excess pattern, bilateral lateral recession is the choice of operation.
ii. In basic exodeviation or the simulated divergence excess pattern combination of recession of lateral rectus with resection of medial rectus of the nondominant eye is the preferred choice.
iii. In case of convergence weakness pattern of exodeviation, bilateral medial recti resection is the operation of choice.

Orthoptic Treatment

If the power of convergence of defective orthoptic exercises to improve this function are indicated. But if convergence spasm. Preoperative orthoptic treatment should be confined to the elimination of suppression and not to the encouragement of convergence.

Preoperative Treatment

If visual acuity of the two eyes is unequal a period of occlusion may be needed in order to equalize it. Treatment to eliminate suppression at the divergent angle may be undertaken as follows:

i. **By exercise with the synoptophore**: Simultaneous perception slides with foveal sized fixation pictures are used.
ii. By teaching the patient to recognize diplopia with the aid of red and green goggles and spot light.

Convergence exercise is not advised preoperatively because over convergence may result postoperatively.

Postoperative Treatment

In the postoperative period orthoptic exercise are advised in order to help maintain comfortable binocular single vision and to improve the range of fusion. Instruments like Ascher Law stereoscope and the diploscope and Remy separator are particularly useful for the post-operative orthoptic exercises. Stereograms may be used for home exercises.

Standard for regarding the patient as orthoptically satisfactory in case of primary exodeviations:

1. The patient should be symptom-free
2. Binocular single vision for near and distance (with or without glasses) should be as good as the uniocular visual acuity of the less efficient eye
3. There should be no manifest deviation. The cover test for near and distance fixation should reveal only a small degree of latent deviation with a rapid recovery to binocular single vision
4. Normal binocular function should be demonstrate with a normal horizontal fusion range
5. Binocular convergence should be well and easily maintained.

MICROFIXATION SYNDROME (MICROTROPIA)

Microstrabismus is also called by the name of retinal slip, fixation disparity, esotropia with fixation disparity, strabismus spurious microtropia unilateral anomalous fusion, microtropia.

As the achievement of binocular single vision in patients with strabismus become more and more important. It became evident that there was a small group of patients with residual strabismus which invited further attention. Then very small angle of deviation (8 prism dioptor or less). They had no diplopia and fusional vergence amplitudes were good microstrabismus is characterized by central suppression.

Scotoma, a very active peripheral binocular vision unharmonious abnormal retinal correspondence was a common finding slight amblyopia.

Patient with unilateral intraocular lesion also had central suppression. They had straight eyes and peripheral fusion. 'Fixation disparity' denote the inexactness of intersection of visual axes at the point of fixation while binocularly fixating. Fixation disparity is a physiologic entity and monofixation syndrome is a pathological one.

In microtropia, there is a high prevalence of anisometropia.

Etiology

Monofixation syndrome:

1. Primary
2. Secondary.

And the presence of central suppression area in the deviated eye:

a. Secondary to strabismus—usually esotropes who have achieved maximum correction, may also be found occasionally in exotropes.
b. Secondary to anisometropia
c. In cases of unilateral macular lesions.

Microbiology

Anisometropia is another etiological factor responsible for disparity in the clarity of images. Bais and fusion predisposes to development of central suppression.

In microtropia—an interesting feature in these patients who show deviation are cover—uncover rest is that the amount of deviation by prism and alternate cover test is greater than that elicited by simultaneous prism and cover test. This is became part of the deviations is made latent by peripheral fusion which is unmasked by alternate cover test. Simultaneous prism and cover test elicits only manifest deviation.

Presence of binocular facultative scotoma is the one constant feature of monofixation syndrome. The scotoma is demonstrated by binocular perimetry in which the two eyes are dissociated with the help of red-green glasses.

Another test that demonstrates this scotoma is the 4 prism diopter (PD) base out prism test. AO vectographic project. O-chart slide also gives a quick means of demonstrating the scotoma.

Diagnostic Method

Besides alternate cover test simultaneous prism and cover test, following are the sensory tests that confirm the diagnosis of monofixation syndrome.

Monofixation Syndrome

1. *Worth form dot-test* **(Fig. 10.16)**. It is done for both near (33 cm) and distance (6 meters). This test often reveals the presence of scotoma and is a quick dated means of evaluating peripheral fusion when done for distance, the dot 3 mm subtend an angle of 1.25° at the nodal point of the eye and for thus near, approximately 6°. A

monofixation is unable to appreciate all four dots at once. He may see only two red or three green dots depending upon the eye affected.

2. When the patient is brought closer to the panel bearing the dots, at one point he begins to appreciate all four dots. It happens at a critical distance, varying with the size of scotoma, as the angle subtended by the dots enlarges sufficiently enough to overcome the area of central suppression. The distance at which this happens allows the indirect estimation of the scotoma size. The latter being inversely proportional to be former.

3. 2.4 PD base out prism test **(Figs 10.17A to D)**. This rest is another method regulating used to reveal the scotoma in patients with monofixation syndrome. In this rest a 4 PD prism is placed base out over one eye, say right, while the patient fixates at a point 6 meters away. The prism displaces the image towards the base, in another words, from the fovea of the right eye to a point outs temporal retina (4 PD or 2° away from the fovea). Refixation movement of the right eye elicits a conjugate movement in the left (Levoversion). If the right eye has no foveal suppression. As consequences of this movement of the left eye the image the image in that eye has been shifted to an extrafoveal point. This eye thus makes a fusional movement back to its original position if foveal suppression is present in that eye, the

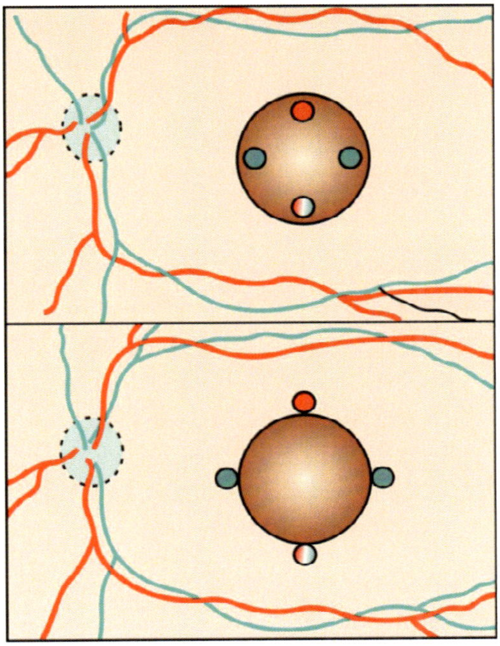

FIG. 10.16: Worth form dot test

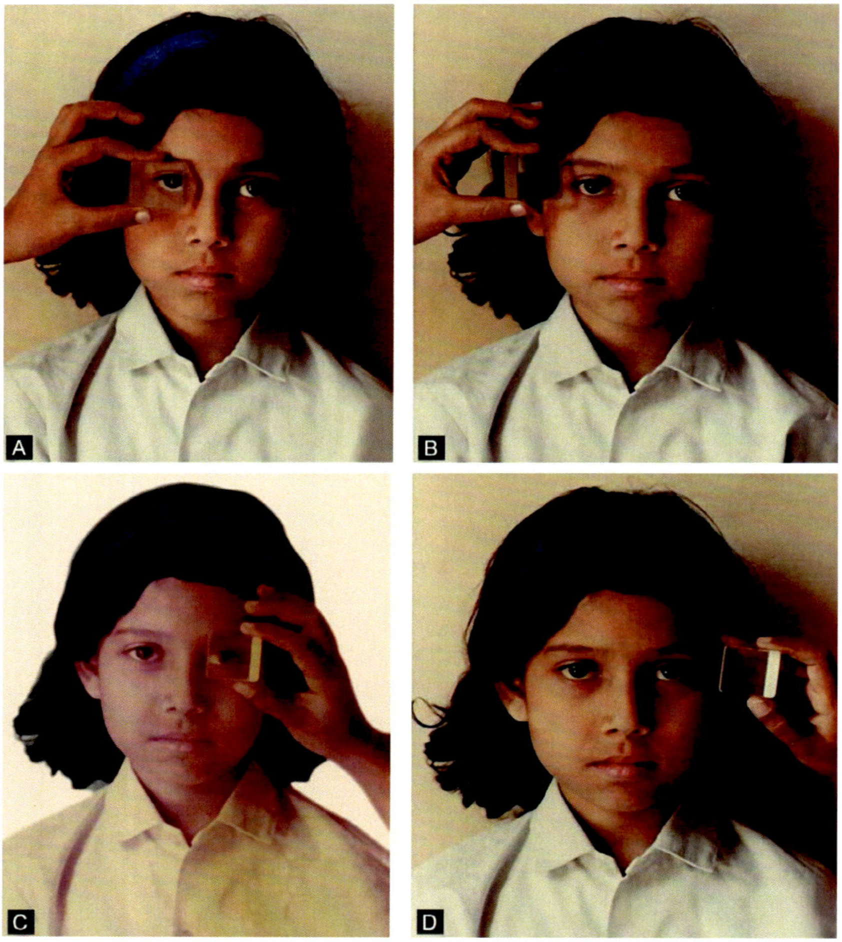

FIGS 10.17A TO D: 4 D prism test in microtropia

fusional movement is absent, however if central suppression is present in the eye which is not covered by the prism. The test is repeated with prism over the left eye. Interpretation of this test is as follows failure of eye with the prism to make a refixation movement or of the follow eye to a fusional movement, indicates the presence of foveal suppression and lack of bifoveal fusion.

Bagolini striated glases test **(Figs 10.18A to C)**: A patient who has a central scotoma in his binocular visual field, will appreciate a break or gap in the streak around the light source. This break is usually ignored unless the patient is made aware of it. Transparency of the glasses has two advantages first, it allows a normal testing environment and second,

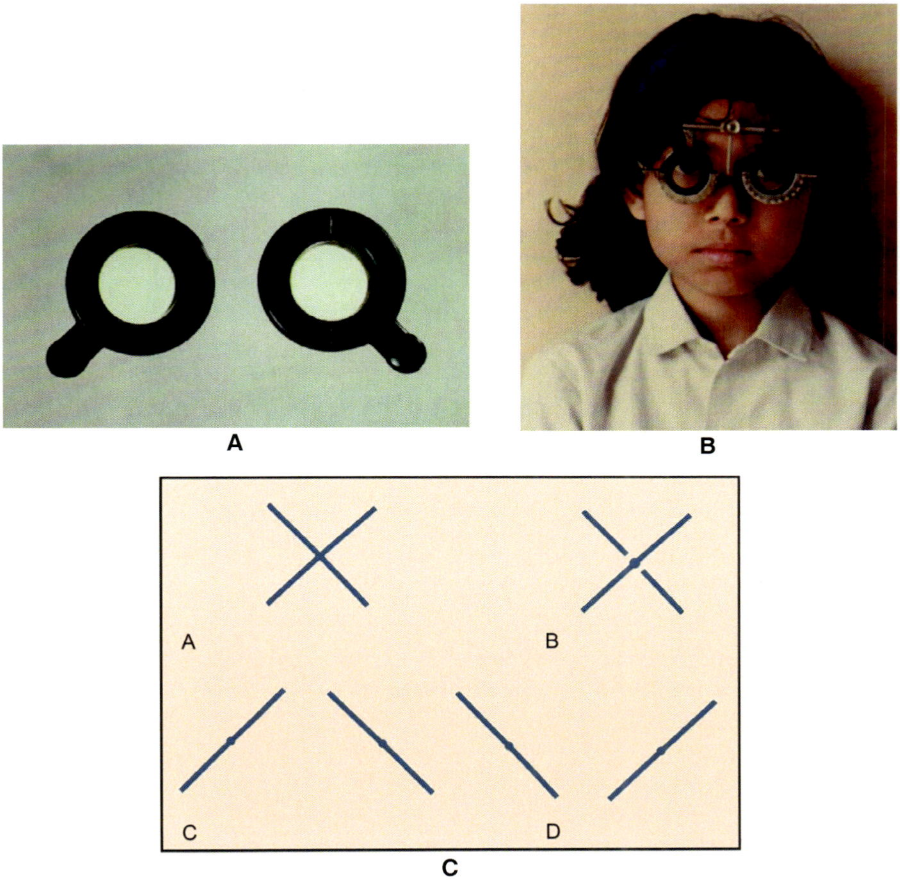

FIG. 10.18A TO C: Bagolini striated test

it allows the examiner to evaluate the alignment of the eyes and the patient's sensorial response, simultaneously. Once the scotoma has been observed in one eye, the patient is encouraged to fixate with the other eye to see if the scotoma has been transferred to the other eye. Bagolini striated glasses test is the best test available for evaluating the status of retinal correspondence in monofixation syndrome.

Treatment of Microtropia

- Treat anisometropia
- Amblyopia is rare, if present, treat the amblyopia
- Iseikonic lens
- Contact lens
- Surgery is not needed.

11 Paralytic Squints

Paralytic squint is that type of squint in which the eyes move in an incoordinated manner so that angle of squint varies in different directions of gaze and on changing fixation from one eye to the other. This is caused by the motor imbalance of one or several extraocular muscles. The characteristic features of the paralytic squint are:

a. A motor deficiency in the field of action of the paretic muscle
b. Diplopia or double vision
c. Secondary deviation is greater than the primary deviation
d. Compensatory head postures
e. Absence of suppression and amblyopia.

ETIOLOGY

Paralysis can be due to:

a. Lesion of the nerve
b. Lesion of the muscles.

Lesion of the nerve can be at the level of nucleus, nerve roots, nerve trunks or it can be a congenital absence or abnormalities of nerve nucleus. It may be due to:

a. Injury
b. Inflammation, e.g. Syphilis, disseminated sclerosis, etc.
c. Vascular diseases, e.g. Hemorrhage, thrombosis aneurysms, arteriosclerosis, etc.
d. Neoplasms, e.g. Brain tumor
e. Toxic, e.g. alcohol, lead, carbon monoxide
f. Degeneration, e.g. Chronic nuclear ophthalmoplegia
g. Other diseases like, thyroid ophthalmoplegia
h. Myasthenia gravis and ocular myopathies
i. Displacement of the visual axis of one eye so that parallelism with that of the other eye is lost. This may occur in:
    1. Injuries like blow out fractures causing damage to the supports of the eyeball.

2. Injuries causing loss of orbital fat such as may be produced by fracture of the floor of the orbit.
3. A space occupying lesion of orbit or adjacent to orbit, e.g. osteoma.

SYMPTOMS

1. *Diplopia* is the chief complaint. It occurs mainly in the field of action of the paralyzed muscle. This could be homonymous or heteronymous **(Figs 11.1A and B)**. In cases of paralysis of long duration and congenital palsy diplopia will not be the chief complaint, since the patient either learns to ignore the false image or contracture of the antagonist increases the deviation so that the false image is thrown on to the less sensitive periphery of retina so that suppression is facilitated.
2. *Vertigo and nausea* is due to diplopia and false orientation. Vertigo occurs mainly when the paralyzed muscle is called into action and is

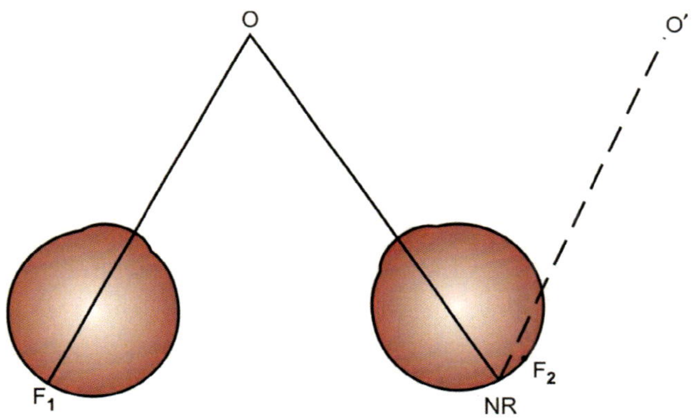

FIG. 11.1A: A Homonymous (uncrossed) diplopia
The image of object O falls on the fovea F1 of the non-deviating eye; and at a point NR nasal to the fovea F2 of the deviating (convergent) eye, the image of O being seen at O′

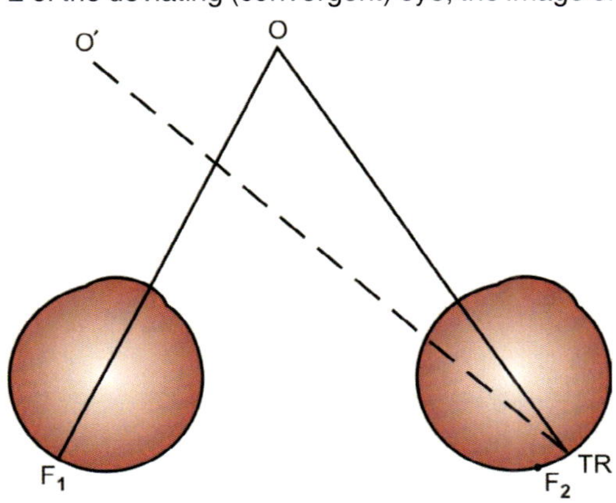

FIGS 11.1B: Heteronomous (crossed) diplopia
The image of object O falls on the fovea F1 of the non-deviating eye; and at a point TR temporal to the fovea F2 of the deviating (divergent) eye, the image of O being seen O′

due to movement of the object with increasing velocity in the direction in which eye is moved.

3. *False projection:* This is a necessary accompaniment of binocular diplopia and depends on the same principle of increase in the secondary deviation, i.e. object is projected according to the amount of nervous energy exerted.
4. *Defective ocular motility:* Limitation of movement in the direction of action of paralyzed muscle is an important feature. The amount of limitation depends on the degree of paralysis.
5. *Complementary head postures:* The purpose of adopting an abnormal head posture is to turn the eyes as far away as possible from the field of action of the paralyzed muscle. This is an attempt to lessen diplopia and associated unpleasant consequences.
   - In dextrorotators (RLR and LMR) palsy the head is turned to right.
   - In SR and IO palsies the chin is elevated.
   - In IR and SO palsies the chin is lowered.

Head tilt—A head tilt to either shoulder, around an anteroposterior axis) may occur to counter act torsional diplopia in paralysis of oblique and vertical muscles. Head tilt is often combined with a head turn and chin elevation or depression and is more common with anomalies of the oblique muscle than the vertical rectus muscles. In short, we can say that head is placed in such a way to avoid action of the affected muscle.

In LSR palsy the head is turned to the left in order to spare the action of the Laevoelevators.

In divergent squints chin is elevated and in convergent squint chin is depressed.

SEQUELAE OF EXTRAOCULAR MUSCLE PALSY (FIG. 11.2)

The paralytic deviation undergoes several stages. The first stage is characterized by weakness of the paretic muscle. Followed by over action of contralateral synergist muscle. Next stages is inhibitory palsy of contralateral antagonist. Occasionally for reasons unknown, the antagonist of the paretic muscle does not over act and the deviation remains limited to the field of action of paretic muscle. For example, (1) In case of RLR palsy. There will be weakness of RLR followed by over action of LMR and there will be contracture of the RMR and secondary inhibitional palsy in LLR. (2) In LSO palsy, there will be weakness of LSO (primary paresin), followed by over action of RIR. Then there will be contracture of LIO and secondary inhibitional palsy of RSR.

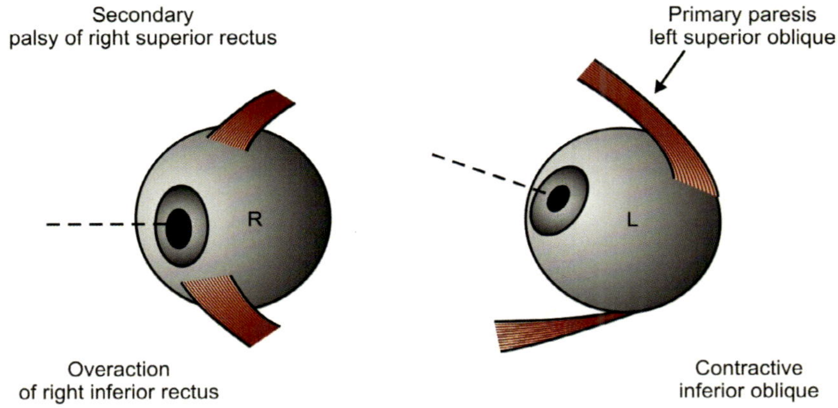

FIG. 11.2: Sequelae of extrinsic ocular muscle palsy

CLINICAL EVALUATION OF THE PATIENT

History

History is most important, from the history we make out the following:

a. Onset is sudden or insidious
b. Presence of diplopia
c. Direction of diplopia
d. History of any other diseases like diabetes, hypertension, multiple sclerosis or malignant diseases especially bronchial carcinoma.

Record of Visual Acuity

If vision is very poor in the affected eye patient may not have diplopia.

Ocular Motility

Record the ocular motility in all the nine positions of gaze. This could be done using a perimeter. Both uniocular and binocular motility should be recorded.

Inspect from Distance

Compensatory Head Postures

The following are the characteristics of head postures:

i. The head is turned into the direction of field of action of the weak muscle so that the eyes are automatically turned into the opposit direction.
ii. Head tilt is to make up for the torsional deviation and is characteristic for the paralysis of oblique.

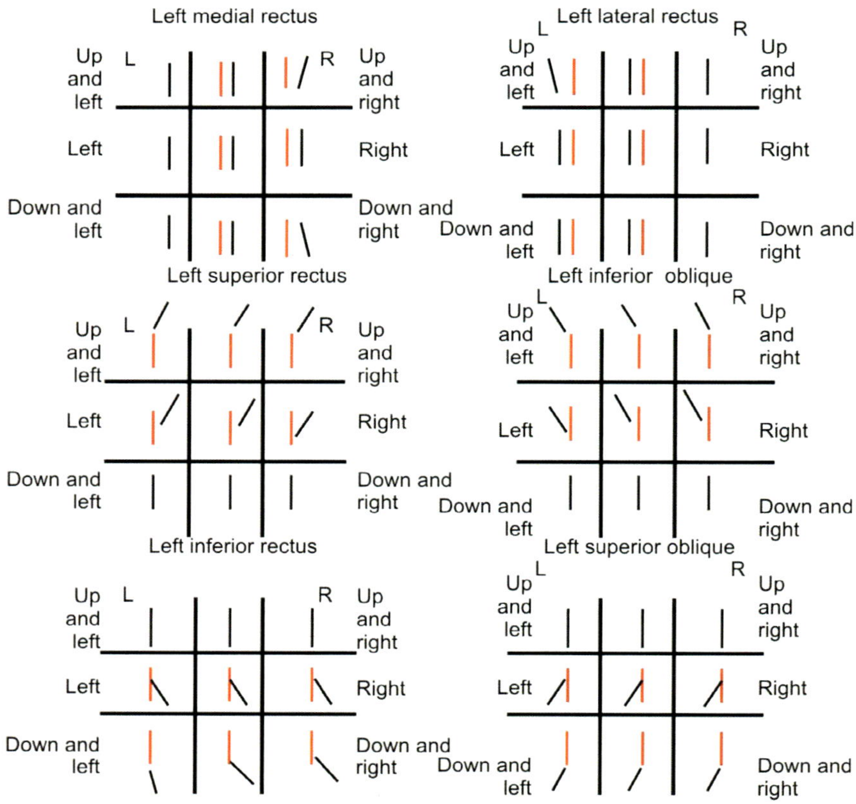

FIG. 11.3: Diplopia charting

Cover Test

In paralytic squint cover test is employed to differentiate primary and secondary deviation. Here secondary deviation is always greater than the primary deviation.

Diplopia Charting (Fig. 11.3)

Diplopia is the most prominent symptoms and very much useful in diagnosis. Carry out the test in a darkroom. Make patient wear Armstrong's glasses. Hold the light at one meter distance from the patient. Hold the light, direct infront of the patient, than move up and down then to right to left, right up, right down, left up an left down, and the positions of the images are accurately recorded on a chart. The following data are derived from the test.

a. The areas of single vision and diplopia
b. Distance between the two images in different areas of diplopia

c. Whether the images are at the same level or not
d. Whether both are erect or one is inclined
e. Whether diplopia is crossed or uncrossed.
N.B. False image belongs to the paralyze eye and distance between the images are maximum in the direction of action of paralyzed muscle.

Hess Charting

This is of both diagnostic and prognostic value.

Advantages

1. Colors of fixation target and indicator are complementary to the goggles.
2. The method is independent of external illumination.
3. It is simple and there cannot be any misinterpretation on the part of the patient or examiner because only one of the red fixation spot light is presented at a time.
4. Less difficulty is encountered in testing patients with gross retinal inhibition as the light source from both fixation object and indicator produce adequate stimulus.

Interpretation

Compare the charts. The smaller chart indicate the paralyzed side and the larger the overacting side. In smaller chart, the greatest restriction indicates the direction of action of paralyzed muscle. In torsional deviations the fields have slopping sides.

Fields of Fixation (Uniocular and Binocular) (Figs 11.4 and 11.5)

a. Field of uniocular fixation in that area within which foveal fixation of a small test object can occur. Its extend corresponds to the limits of movements of the eyeball in different direction. This could be measured by means of a perimeter. The extend of field in the average normal eye is about 45°–50° except in the inner and downwards where it is limited to some extent by nose.
b. The fields of binocular fixation is that area within which bifoveal fixation of a small test object can occur. Its extent is limited partly by the limits of ocular movements and partly by nose. For the test to be of value the patients cooperation must be good and his binocular vision is strong. The test objects usually employed is 3-5 mm size and color is white.

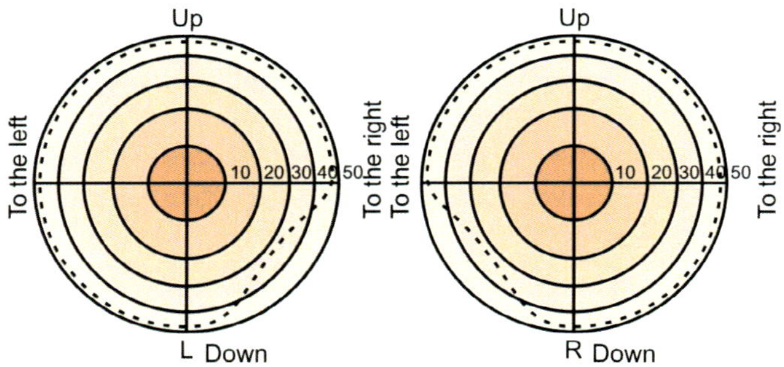

FIG. 11.4: Field of uniocular fixation

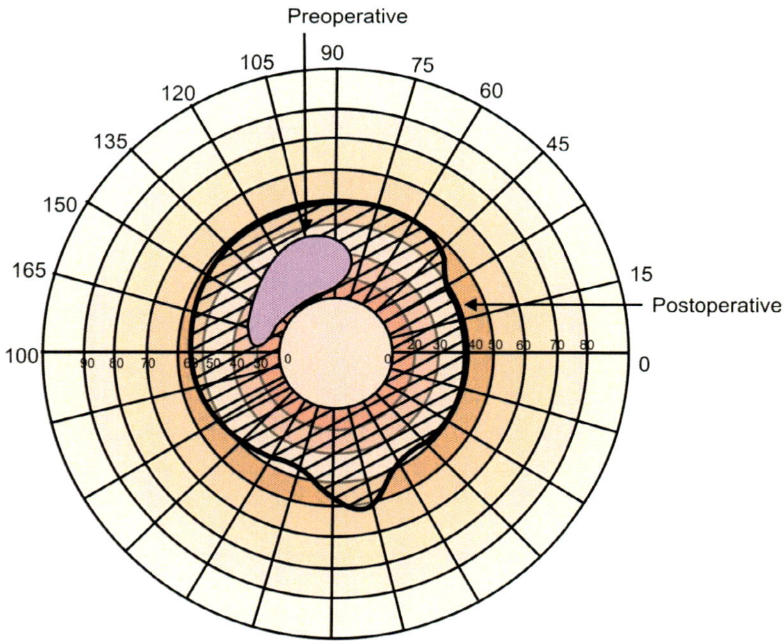

FIG. 11.5: Field of binocular fixation

Bielschowky's Head Tilt Test

Bielschowky's head tilt test is of great value in diagnosing paresis of the oblique muscle than that of rectus muscle because the vertical effect of obliques, provoked by tilting the head to either shoulder in patients with paralysis of vertical rectus muscle is less than that of rectus muscle.

Routine Ophthalmoscopic Examination

Routine ophthalmoscopic examination especially to study the disk for papilledema or papillitis.

Forced Duction Test

This test is performed by anesthetizing the conjunctiva over the insertion of the muscle to be tested. Grasp the insertion of the muscle with a toothed forceps and attempt to rotate the eye in the field of action of weak muscle.

This is of great value in deciding whether the anomaly of ocular motility is caused by mechanical factor such as contracture or fibrosis of a muscle, tightness of muscle following excessive resection, and shrinkage and scarring of the conjunctiva or Tenon's capsule.

Estimation of Generated Muscle Force

This test is helpful to judge the residual function of an apparently paretic muscle. The active force generate by muscle can be estimated by stabilizing the eye with a forceps while the patient moves his eyes against the resistance. The tug that examiner feels on the forceps is a sign of residual function. Absence of the tug is a sign of complete paralysis.

Exaggerated Force Duction Test

It is to estimate the tightness of oblique muscle. For this test eye must be put in the orbit (retroplace the globe) as it is then rocked back and forth by extorting and moving the globe around the tendon to check the tight oblique muscle now.

Differential Intraocular Pressure

The generated muscle could be estimated by comparing into ocular pressure in various positions of gazes and pressure increases as may be as high as 50 mm kg in case of restrictive elements.

Eye Movement Velocity

It may be useful only as an auxiliary diagnostic method, in evaluating the paralytic squint the eyes are capable of morning saccades/first eye movements upto the velocity of 200–5000/sec. In cases of paralysis slow drifting eye movement, restriction squints have normal saccadic velocity till the restriction comes into effect.

Electromyography

Electromyography is useful procedure to test the function of each muscle separately and follow-up study will indicates whether the muscle is in the process of recovery or not.

Electro-oculography

Electro-oculography is an auxiliary diagnostic method.

Doll's Head Phenomenon

Doll's head phenomenon is tested by turning the head in different directions and noting the movement of the eye. This is an important evidence for the intactness of the oculomotor nucleus in patient with supranuclear paralysis.

Bell's Phenomenon

Where in the eyes move upwards on forcible closure of the lids may be of diagnostic importance. For its presence the brainstem pathways must be intact even although the frontal bulbar pathway is disrupted. It occur in peripheral fascial palsy in which the lid fail to close when the patient attempts to close the eyes, the lids on the paralyzed side fail to shut and a slight upward movement of globe is observed, Bell's phenomenon is absent in nuclear lesion of the 7th cranial nerve which lends support to the theory that reflex is mediated through lower centers, probably by way of the posterior longitudinal bundle.

Neurological Examination

It is important to determine whether the palsy is nuclear supranuclear and whether there is any focus of irritation or pressure in the course of the nerve involved.

Special Tests

Prostigmine/Neostigmine test to rule out myasthenia in cases of transient and intermittent squints.

Investigations for Thyroid Functions

Investigations for thyroid functions, whenever relevant to rule out thyroid ophthalmoplegia.

Testing of Corneal Sensation

Testing of corneal sensation is also done whenever necessary.

Other Investigations

a. Investigations for systemic diseases like diabetes, hypertension, syphilis, etc.

b. X-ray skull
c. X-ray sinus and orbit
d. X-ray chest
e. Complete hemogram
f. CT scanning to ultrasonography
g. Carotid angiography
h. Orbital venography.

TYPES OF PARALYSIS

Depending on the involvement of individual muscles or group of muscles there can be many form of paralysis.

The main are as follows:

IIIrd Nerve Palsy

a. Complete third nerve palsy — Here only spared muscles are lateral rectus and superior oblique. The eye will be depressed, abducted and intorted. LPS paralysis, causes ptosis as well. In complete IIIrd nerve palsy the intrinsic muscles are also involved causing dilatation of pupil and loss of accommodation.
b. Isolated paralysis of individual muscle, i.e. SR, MR, IR or IO do occur, though rarely.

IVth Nerve Palsy

The movement affected are adduction and depression, superior oblique being the muscle paralyzed. The eye may be hypertropic due to over action of the antagonist. Head will be tilted to the normal side and chin will be depressed. Patients with bilateral SO palsy will have right hypertropia in left gaze and left hypertropia in right gaze, which increases on tilting the head on either sides.

VIth Nerve Palsy

Adduction will be affected, lateral rectus being the muscle paralyzed. The palpebral fissure may be widened on looking to the side of paralysis (adduction), due to maximal innervational effort. Esotropia may be present in the primary position. Head is turned over the affected shoulder.

Pseudograefe Sign

During the recovery of the IIIrd nerve palsy, nerve fibers originally connected with inferior ractus grow into the sheath of nerves fibers supplying the levator muscle so that impulse to look down increase the tonus of the levator, hence there will be retraction of the upper lid in downward gaze, it may be accompanied by contraction of the pupil.

MANAGEMENT

Treatment of paralytic squint is always difficult and must depend on casual conditions. Every case of paralytic squint should be managed initially on conservations lines.

The Indications for Therapy

1. Presence of diplopia in the practical field of fixation
2. Inability to maintain binocular single vision without anomalous head posture.

Prisms are effective in treating deviations less than 10. for larger deviations prisms are not usually tolerated for prolonged periods and in such cases surgery becomes unavoidable. Fresnel prisms are tried, but it should be kept in mind that the prisms take away whatever stimulus left to control strabisms and this may eventually lead to an increase in the extent of residual deviation.

Treatment of Diplopia

Management of diplopia in a case awaiting spontaneous recovery or surgery is important.

If the patient does not have BSV in any position of gaze simple eye shields are given to cover each eye alternately.

If the patient enjoys BSV in certain gazes the occlusion need not be complete, but it may be so arranged that BSV may be exercised in a limited area, i.e. occlude part of the field of one eye only.

Orthoptic treatment to maintain simultaneous binocular vision, and prevention of suppression is of almost importance.

Surgical Correction

The aim of the surgery in a case of paralytic squint is to abolish diplopia and to regain comfortable binocular vision in all directions of gaze as well as to produce a good cosmetic look. Operation is delayed until 6 months since the onset of deviation in order to allow spontaneous recovery and to stabilize the squint.

Surgical Procedures

Surgery for VIth Nerve Palsy

Sixth nerve palsy can be unilateral or bilateral. It can be aparesis or paralysis.

In unilateral palsy

1. See whether contracture is fully developed or not.
2. Assess the deviation for near and distance.
   i. If the muscle sequent has fully developed, the angle of deviation is same on dextroversion and on levoversion. In such cases you will have to do a resection of LR along with recession of the ipsilateral MR. However if the angle of deviation is small resection of LR alone may be sufficient.
   ii. If the muscle sequelae is partially developed, i.e. there is no contracture of the MR but there is over action of the contralateral MR in such cases you will have to do LR resection along with recession of the contralateral MR or alternately a Faden operation:
      1. Here the rectus muscle is first recessed and muscle belly is anchored to the sclera by one or more circumferentially placed mattress sutures. The muscle is then reinserted in its original position.
      2. The muscle remain inserted. The edges of the muscle are attached to the globe. The appropriate distance of posterior fixation sutures behind the normal muscle insertion is MR 11-13 mm.

         In this procedure the power of the muscle is decreased although its primary position is not altered.
   iii. In the case of VIth nerve palsy and the eye is not moving even upto midline, see whether it is a case o MR contracture or complete loss of function of LR.

This is feasible by:

(i) Forced duction test
(ii) Forced generation test
(iii) EMG
(iv) EOG, etc.

If there is MR contracture with LR function, in such cases, do resection of the LR along with recession of MR.

In case of contracture of MR with no LR function recess MR at least 7 mm with recession of overlying conjunctiva. A transposition operation (reverse Jensens) is also indicated.

In bilateral palsy: It is usual to operate first on the nonfixing eye followed by surgey on the fixing eye at a second stage some weeks later.

In the case of both VIth and IIIrd nerve palsy the VIth nerve palsy should be treated first (as outlined in Table 11.1).

IVth Nerve Palsy

In IVth nerve palsy the choice of surgery depends on:

1. Whether the palsy is unilateral or bilateral
2. Whether the sequelae have developed particularly whether there is overaction of the inferior oblique
3. The presence and amount of extorsion and whether this is superable.

In unilateral palsy: The surgery is usually performed and on overacting muscle, not on the superior oblique itself, because of technical difficulties, and plication on the vertical component is unpredictable as compared to the effect on cyclodeviation. There is also likelihood of inducing Brown's syndrome.

If the muscle sequelae has fully developed, there will be overaction of the contralateral inferior rectus, contracture of the inferior oblique and secondary underaction of the superior rectus. Vertical deviation will be same on contralateral up gaze and down gaze. Weakening of IO is the operation of choice.

If torsion is insuperable, recession of IR is contraindicated and a Harada procedure on the affected superior oblique should be performed as a first stage.

According to Payman the surgery to the VIth nerve palsy depends on the degree of abduction possible (Table 11.1).

Divergence paralysis: May be difficult to differentiate from unilateral or bilateral VIth nerve palsy, but this condition is usually comitant. The esotropia is unchanged or may decrease on lateroversion, unlike without a VIth nerve palsy, fusional divergence amplitudes are either severally reduced or absent, causes are head trauma intracranial space occupying lesions and cerebrovascular accidents.

Harada procedure: The anterior half of the superior oblique tendon is disinserted and split from the posterior portion along the line of its

TABLE 11.1: Surgery for lateral rectus palsies

Almost full abduction	5° (10Δ) Esotropia in primary position—10 mm Resection of paretic LR muscle
More or equal	5° (10Δ) Eso in primary position – (a) 10 mm Resection of paretic LR (b) 5 mm recession of antagonistic MR
(In another case) Limited abduction can abduct beyond midline	≤ 16° (32Δ) Eso in primary position (a) 8-10 mm Resection of LR muscle (b) 5mm recession antagonist MR mus
	> 16° (32Δ) Eso in primary position (a) 8-10 mm resection of LR muscle (b) 5 mm recession antagonist MR muscle (c) 5 mm recession of Yoke MR muscle
Limited abduction cannot abduct to midline	5 mm recession of MR (a) along with recession of conjunctiva over MR (b) Resect 10 mm LR If passive abduction is limited recess MR another 3-5 mm. At the end of surgery, full passive rotation must be possible

fibers for some 10mm. The mobilized portion is then reattached 8 mm. Posterior to LR insertion and just above the LR muscles upper margin.

Once the torsion has been reduce, the vertical deviation can be reassessed and contralateral inferior rectus recessed.

In bilateral SO palsy, i.e. when there is:

1. Insuperable torsion – (torsional diplopia)
2. The head posture is mainly one of chin depression
3. Only a small vertical deviation in primary position.

Here bilateral Harada operation is the most effective procedure to overcome torsional deviation. If the palsy is asymmetrical maximum amount is performed on the more affected side and a smaller amount of the other eye. Further surgery may be necessary to correct a residual vertical deviation.

If there is marked contracture of both IO. Bilateral weakening surgery on the muscles is the first choice. Further surgery depends on the effect on cyclodeviation.

The 'V' pattern if marked need to be considered, either during vertical muscle surgery at a later stage.

IIIrd Nerve Palsy

Complete paralysis: In a case of complete IIIrd nerve palsy with contracture of the two remaining active muscles, i.e. SO and LR weakening procedures are adopted.

1. LR recession by 10mm with recession of the overlying conjunctiva.
2. SO tenectomy—this helps to avoid mechanically induced hypotropia.

Strengthening procedures—A superomaximal (up to 8 mm) resection of MR.

Alternatively—Muscle transportion procedures like Jenson's procedure are also indicated.

In paresis—It is advisable to correct the horizontal angle initially by resection of MR and recession of LR residual deviation can be treated conservatively with prisms or by surgery to strengthen the SR or IR.

COMPLETE PARALYSIS OR PARESIS

a. **Medial rectus**—Resection of MR with ipsilateral or contralateral LR recession.
b. **Inferior rectus palsy**—Resection of IR and ipsilateral SR recession.
c. **Superior rectus palsy**—Resection of SR weakening of the IR and IO
d. **Inferior oblique palsy**—Intrasheath tenotomy of ipsilateral SO, a recession of the contralateral SR depending whether the hypotropia is more marked in down gaze and on the amount of torsional deviation.

Weakening Operation

Recession (Rectus muscle weakening operation).

Hang back recession—In this method muscle is disinserted and reattached to its original insertion.

BLOWOUT FRACTURE

A blunt injury to the eye causes increased orbital pressure, and the orbit tends to give way at its weakest point, the orbital floor. As a result, the ligament of Lockwood drops down and the inferior rectus and occasionally the inferior oblique are trapped in the fracture. Limitation of action of the superior and inferior rectus muscles and occasionally the inferior ethmoidal area may cause simultaneous limitation of lateral rotation. There may also be a relative enophthalmos, or this may develop later as the edema surrounding the fracture subsides or as the orbital fat atrophies. Damage to the infraorbital nerve with anesthesia of the lower lid and cheek can occur. The eyes be straight in the primary position, or the patient may have a hypotropia with diplopia in the up and down positions because of the superior and inferior rectus muscles restrictions.

Ocular Myopathy

This is a progressive external ophthalmoplegia. There is limitation of extra- ocular movement and progressive ptosis ultimately the patient ends up with a total ophthalmoplegia (it is not usually necessary to perform surgery on the extraocular muscles because the patient's eyes are straight in the primary position).

Myasthenia Gravis

Myasthenia gravis is a disease characterized by fatigue and weakness of striated muscles within the body. This is due to blockage at the neuro-muscular end plate, symptoms of ocular myasthenia gravis include diplopia and ptosis symptoms of myasthenia gravis are less in the morning and they are worse towards the end of the day when patient become fatigued. Diagnosis is confirmed in most cases by the administration of tensilon intravenously see if there is any improvement in clinical signs or symptoms, tonography is useful on making the diagnosis.

Painful Ophthalmoplegia

Refer to the involvement of one of more of the ocular motor nerves by a chronic granulomatous or nongranulomatous inflammation, usually at the orbital apex, in the superior orbital tissues, or in the cavernosus sinus patient experience pain and involvement of IIIrd, IVth and VIth nerve. If the orbital apex is involved, there may be visual loss from involvement of the optic nerve ESR is usually high. Many terms have been used to describe the syndrome, including the orbital apex syndrome, superior orbital fissure syndrome and Tolosa Hunt syndrome.

DOUBLE ELEVATOR PALSY

Double elevator palsy is a common of hyperdeviation. There is a parises of the superior rectus and inferior oblique muscles in the same eye. The inferior oblique shows more restriction than superior rectus. Ptosis and occasionally Marcus Gunn (Jaw winking) may also be associated. The patient will generally walk with the head elevating slightly in order to maintain binocular vision just below the midline and in the inferior field of gaze.

Double elevator palsy probably results from some type of congenital nuclear lesion, because in the orbit the superior rectus and medial rectus.

Marcus Gunn phenomenon is apparently caused by misdirected nerve pathway. In cases with ptosis, surgery for have a risk of exposure Bell's phenomenon.

Treatment

Surgery is the main stay of treatment in such cases. However, no surgery is indicated if the patient has binocular vision in a straight ahead position, deviation showing only on locking up and there is no backward head tilt in the primary position.

The surgical approach depends upon the amount of elevation achieved in the affected eye can be elevated above the midline the procedure of choice is to weaken yoke muscles, that is, the superior rectus and inferior oblique muscle in the normal eye. The superior rectus 4-5 mm and the inferior oblique 8- mm. In cases where the eye cannot be brought above the midtime recession of IR and resection SR muscle in the affected eye is required. In some of the patient who had undergone surgery on MR for esotropia, the eye develop a market esotropia and the patient tries to elevate the eye. In the down gaze, the same patient has a large esotropia. The eye cannot be elevated to midtime in either the adducted or abducted position. Because if this limitation, the condition has been called "congenital fibroses syndrome. Such eyes require recession of IR and congenital, the SR is reseated 4-5 mm.

Differential Diagnosis of Ocular vs Congenital Torticollis (Tables 11.2 and 11.3)

The cause of congenital (nonocular) torticollis include:

a. Congenital bony malformations of Atlas (Atlas = Ist vertebra), cervical vertebrae and ribs.
b. Malformation of sternomastoid muscles.

TABLE 11.2: Difference between ocular and congenital torticollis

Ocular Torticollis	Congenital torticollis
1. —	1. Marked resistance to passive straightening of the head
2. —	2. Often, a fibroma mass may be felt in the contracted sternomastoid muscle
3. Patching (occlusion) of the paretic muscle can relive ocular torticollis, provided no secondary) skeletal or muscular changes have developed in the neck	3. Patching has no effect on congenital torticollis

TABLE 11.3: Differential diagnosis between congenital and acquired palsy

Congenital	Acquired
1. Intermittent diplopia	(A)
2. Intermittent squint	(A)
3. Head posture but patient is unaware of this	(A)
4. Anatomical changes in vertebral column	(A)
5. Suppression is usually present	(A)

TOTAL OPHTHALMOPLEGIA

Inv. of Extrinsic, ocular muscle
Intrinsic ocular muscle
IPS
Ptosis+
Proptosis+

Ocular movement (A) or restricted
Pupillary activity to light
Accommodation and convergence (A)

DOUBLE DEPRESSOR PARALYSIS

Double depressor paralysis is a rare anomaly and it consists of inability to depress the eye from primary position, adduction or abduction. This is caused by long-standing paralysis of the inferior rectus muscle rather by paralysis of both inferior rectus and superior oblique muscle (Table 11.4).

Botulinum Toxin

In paralytic strabismus, the botulinum induced paralysis of the antagonist muscle prevents or reduces its contracture during spontaneous recovery of the paretic muscle. Also, as the initial overaction resulting from the injection slowly resolves and the eyes approach the primary position, fusion may "lock on" resulting in Orthophora.

TABLE 11.4: Differential diagnosis between paralytic and nonparalytic squint

Paralytic	*Nonparalytic*
1. Eyes move in such an incoordinated manner so that the angle of squint varies in different direction of gazes and on changing fixation from one to other eye.	1. Eyes move in coordinated manner and angle of squint remain same in all direction of gaze
2. Diplopia is a prominent feature	2. No. diplopia
3. Nausea and vertigo	3. (A)
4. Compensatory head posture	4. (A)
5. Onset – sudden	5. Usually in children
6. Amblyopia, supervision, ARC, eccentric fixation absent	6. Amblyopia, supervision, ARC, eccentric fixation present
7. Secondary deviation/primary deviation	7. Secondary = Primary deviation
8. Some changes present in uninvolved muscle	8. Not so
9. Palliative treatment is required	9. No palliative treatment
10. Wait for 6-8 months for surgery	10. Immediate it is required

The advantages of botulinum toxin therapy for strabismus are: (1) it can be performed on an outpatient basis, (2) it carries minimum risk, (3) leaves no scar, (4) can be used for postoperative residual strabismus and (5) can be used when surgery is inappropriate. It has been shown in paralytic strabismus toxin have better chance of recovery than those that have not been treated. In lateral rectus palsy contacture of the antagonist medial rectus muscle can be prevented and this should make subsequent elective surgery easier.

The disadvantages of botulinum toxin therapy for strabismus are: (1) more than two injection is often needed to determine the optimum dose to obtain maximal benefit, (2) alignment changes are not as stable as with surgery and (3) transient partial ptosis and vertical strabismus frequently occur. There is dramatic relief of symptoms following treatment with botulinum toxin.

The other reported complication of botulinum therapy are: (1) scleral perforation, (2) retrobulbar hemorrhages, (3) diplopia, (4) pupillary dilatation, (5) ecchynosis, (6) corneal exposure, (7) ptosis, (8) ectropon, (9) lagophthalmos and (10) chemosis.

Botulinum toxin is curative in some cases of paralytic strabismus, in others it prevent contracture of the antagonist and should therefore make subsequent surgery simple.

APPLIED ANATOMY

Oculomotor Nerve (IIIrd N) (Fig. 12.6)

The oculomotor or the IIIrd cranial nerve innervates all the extraocular muscles except the lateral rectus and the superior oblique. In addition, it carries the parasympathetic fibers to the ciliary muscle and the sphincter pupillae. The nucleus of IIIrd nerve is in the form of a complex formed by a number of subnuclei and is situated in the midbrain) at the level of superior colliculi. Below the aqueduct of Sylvius. The subnuclei include:

i. *Subnucleus for levator*: It lies in the caudal part of the complex and is unpaired, thus supplying levator muscle of the lids of both eyes. Therefore, a lesion confined to this area will lead to ptosis of both eyes.

ii. *Subnucleus for superior rectus*: This is paired, and supplies the contralateral superior rectus muscle. This implies that in a case of IIIrd nerve palsy, if the contralateral superior rectus has been spared, the lesion does not lie in the nucleus.

iii. *Subnucleus for medial rectus, inferior rectus and inferior oblique*: This is also a paired group of cells, supplying the corresponding muscles of the same (ipsilateral) side.

iv. *Accessory nucleus*: Situated posterior to the main mass, it sends preganglionic parasympathetic fibers along the motor fibers, and is related to the phenomenon of near reflex, accommodation, and perhaps, convergence (Perlia's nucleus).

In general, it is rare to see lesions purely localized in the nuclear complex. Certain vascular lesion, demyelinating diseases and tumors may involve this region.

The efferent fibers from the complex form the fasciculus, which travel through the red nucleus and medial part of the cerebral peduncles, emerging from midbrain. Lesions in this zone are caused by the same conditions as in the case of nuclear complex, and may lead to two well-recognized syndromes:

Benedikt's syndrome: This is characterized by an ipsilateral IIIrd nerve palsys and a contralateral hemiplegia with tremors. This is the result of lesions of the fasciculus in the red nucleus.

Weber's syndrome: This caused by the fascicular lesion in the cerebral peduncles, and is characterized by an ipsilateral IIIrd nerve palsy accompanied by a contralateral hemiparesis.

The basilar part of the nerve is constituted by 15-20 rootlets in the interpeduncular area which join one another to form the main trunk.

The main trunk of the nerve is flattened at the beginning, twists around to bring the inferior fibers superiorly and assumes a rounded shape. It travels between the posterior cerebral and superior cerebellar arteries. Further forwards, it lies lateral and parallel to the posterior communicating artery, reaching the cavernous sinus. During this course, as it traverses the base of skull, it is unaccompanied by any other cranial nerve. It is, therefore, quite common to see isolated palsy of the third nerve in the basilar part, caused by aneurysms or head injuries.

A painful IIIrd nerve palsy with pupillary involvement is typically seen in the aneurysms at the junction of the posterior communicating artery and the internal carotid artery **(Fig. 11.6)**.

In a case of extradural hematoma following head injury, a pressure may result leading to herniation of the temporal lobe. This compresses the third nerve over the tentorial edge, manifesting initially as a dilated and fixed pupil followed by a total palsy of the nerve.

The intracavernous part, the nerve enters the cavernous sinus by piercing the dura in its posterior part just lateral to the posterior clinoid processes, lying superior to the trochlear nerve.

In the anterior part, it divides into superior and inferior division and enters the orbit via the middle portion of superior orbital fissure within the annulus of Zinn.

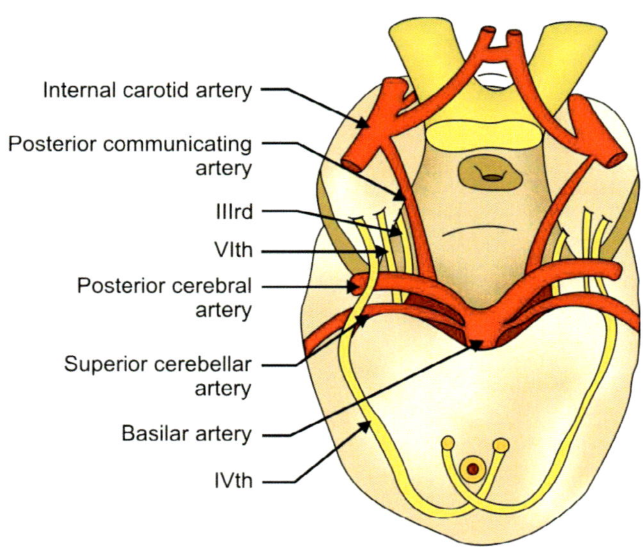

FIG. 11.6: Anatomy of IIIrd nerve

Cavernous sinus lesions such as aneurysms, carotidcavernous fistula, Tolosa-Hunt syndrome may cause IIIrd nerve palsy in association with palsy of other nerves within the cavernous sinus, i.e. the IVth nerve and the first division of Vth nerve. The pupil usually remains unaffected. Diabetes is another important condition that may cause a vascular palsy of the IIIrd nerve.

The intraorbital part, the nerve enters the orbit after dividing into a superior division (supplying the levator and superior rectus), and inferior division (supplying medial rectus, inferior rectus and inferior oblique) muscles. The inferior division also carries parasympathetic fibers from Edinger-Westphal nucleus to sphincter pupillae and the ciliary muscle.

The nature of blood supply to the third nerve has important clinical bearings. While the pupillomotor fibers located in the median and superior part of the third nerve is nourished by the pial vessels, the main trunk derives its blood via vasa nervosum. The surgical conditions like aneurysms and head injury compress the pial vessels leading to the paralysis of pupillomotor fibers. On the other hand, medical conditions like diabetes and hypertension primarily affect the vasa nervosum and so, the pupillomotor fibers may be spared **(Fig. 11.7).**

THE TROCHLEAR NERVE (IVTH N)

This is the longest and the thinnest of all cranial nerves. It is purely a motor nerve innervating the superior oblique muscle of the opposite side. It is also peculiar in that it emerges out from the dorsal aspect of the brain.

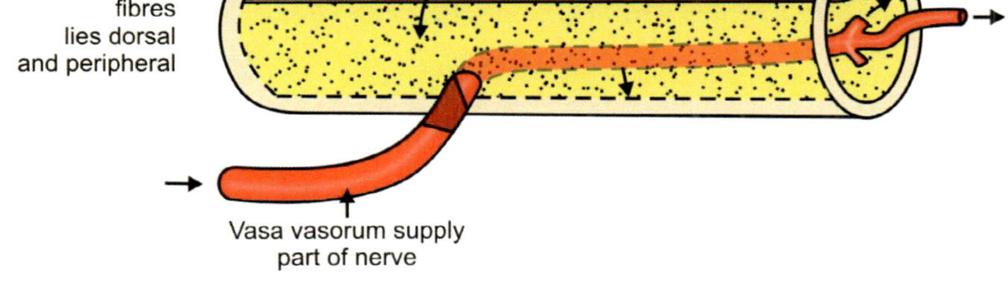

FIG. 11.7: Location of pupillomotor fibres in IIIrd nerve

The nucleus of trochlear nerve lies in the midbrain at the level of inferior colliculi, and is in continuation with the nucleus of IIIrd nerve.

The fascicular component is constituted by the axons that curve around the aqueduct of Sylvius and decussate completely.

The trunk (precavernous part), emerges on the dorsal aspect of the midbrain and curves forward between the posterior cerebral and the superior cerebellar runs arteries as does the trunk of IIIrd nerve. It pierces the dura below the IIIrd nerve to enter the posterior part of cavernous sinus. The infracavernous part lies in the lateral wall of the sinus below the third nerve and above the first division of Vth nerve. In the anterior part, it crosses over the IIIrd nerve and enters the orbit through lateral part of the superior orbital fissure, superotemporal to the annulus of Zinn.

The intraorbital part carries the nerve supply to the superior oblique muscle.

THE ABDUCENS NERVE (VITH N)

The VIth cranial nerve is motor in function, has a long course and innervates the lateral rectus muscle of the same side.The nucleus of sixth nerve lies in the middle of pons below the fourth ventricle and is closely associated with the fasciculus of the facial nerve. In addition, it is also connected with the pretectal nucleus of both sides as well as the horizontal gaze center in the pontine paramedial reticular formation. Therefore, any lesion affecting the zone of VIth nerve. Nucleus will not cause an isolated paralysis of the ipsilateral lateral rectus muscle, but will be accompanied by:

i. Paralysis of conjugate movements towards the side of lesion
ii. Ipsilateral facial nerve palsy, by way of the involvement of fasciculus of facial nerve.

The fascicular part is composed of the axons emerging from the nucleus, pass forwards through the medial meniscus and the pyramidal tract leaving the brainstem at the junction of pons and midbrain, lateral to the pyramidal prominence. In view of its course through the pyramidal tract and medial meniscus. A lesion in the region of fascicule is likely to cause multiple clinical manifestations in the form of Foville's syndrome. This is manifested if the lesion is located at the site where the fasciculus traverses the medial meniscus, and shows:

- Paralysis of the ipsilateral lateral rectus muscle, paralysis of the lateral gaze

- Paralysis of the lateral gaze towards the same side
- Facial weakness (damage to the facial nerve nucleus)
- Facial analgesia (damage to the sensory portion of Vth nerve)
- Homer's syndrome
- Deafness.

Millard-Gubler syndrome. The lesion at the sight of the fasciculus passing through the pyramidal tract will be characterized by paralysis of the ipsilateral lateral rectus muscle.

Contralateral Hemiplegia

The basilar portion of the nerve, after emerging from the pontomedullary junction, passes upwards close to the base of the pons and is crossed by the anterior inferior cerebellar artery. It runs further upwards on the back of petrous temporal bone near its apex turning sharply at right angle on the sharp border of the petrous bone before piercing the dura to enter the cavernous sinus, lateral to the dorsum sellae. Damage to the basilar portion may occur in the following situations:

i. *Acoustic neuroma*: This tumor located at the cerebellopontine angle may cause damage to multiple cranial nerves, *viz.* the Vth, VIth, VIIth, and VIIIth nerves. Therefore, paralysis of the lateral rectus in such cases is accompanied by a hearing loss which is the first symptom, and loss of corneal sensation which is the first sign (i.e. it precedes the VIth nerve involvement).

ii. *Nasopharyngeal tumors*: Following the invasion of skull and its foramina, these tumors can damage the VIth nerve in it basilar course.

iii. *Raised intracranial pressure* **(Fig. 11.8):** The increased pressure, especially in case of posterior fossa tumors or in benign intracranial hypertention (pseudotumor cerebri) tends to push the brain downwards. Such a movement may damage the VIth nerve on stretching at the sharp border of petrous bone where it makes a sharp right angled turn. The nerves may be damaged on both the sides. The resultant VIth nerve palsy, however, has no localizing value.

iv. *Basal skull fracture*: Damage to the VIth nerve (unilateral or bilateral) in this situation is nonspecific, and may be a part of the overall damage to the brain tissue.

The infracavernous part of the nerve lies below the IIIrd and IVth nerve, as well as the first division of the Vth nerve, placed most medially

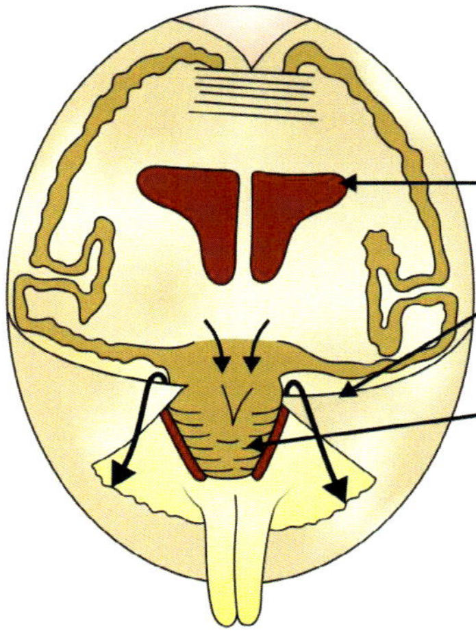

Fig. 11.8: Mechanism of bilateral VIth nerve palsy resulting from raised intraocular pressure

and close to the internal carotid artery, thus rendering it more vulnerable than other nerves. It also carries the sympathetic fibers from the para-carotid plexus and thus a paralysis of the intracavernous portion of the nerve may be associated with a postganglionic Homer syndrome (Parkinson sign).

The nerve gets involved by the same set of lesions involving the IIIrd and the IVth nerve inside the cavernous sinus.The infraorbital part of the nerve begins with its entry to the orbit through the annulus of Zinn, and innervates the lateral rectus muscle.

12 Vertical Strabismus

As in the case of horizontal deviations, a vertical squint can be concomitant or incomitant (congenital or acquired). It may express itself in the form of a hyperphoria, intermittent hypertropia, or a (constant) hypertropia. Depending upon the eye involved, it may be right hypertropia or left hypertropia.

COMITANT VERTICAL DEVIATIONS

It is not uncommon to see such type of deviations, either in an isolated form or in association with horizontal deviations. The underlying cause is not well-understood. Some form of innervational disturbance may be a likely factor. In many instances, it may be the result of a paralytic incomitant hyperdeviation attaining the character of a comitant deviation over a long period of time. The common features of such deviations are as follows:

i. Intermittent hypertropia is more common than a constant deviation
ii. Suppression, amblyopia or a vertical anomalous retinal correspondence may be present
iii. Small vertical deviations are typically present in association with moderate to large horizontal deviations
iv. Many cases demonstrate an under or over action of one or more cyclovertical muscles.

Treatment

Orthoptic treatment is directed to treat amblyopia. In small deviations upto 15 prism diopters, prisms are provided to neutralize the deviation. The power of prism is equally divided in two eyes with the base down in front of the hypertropic eye and base up in the other eye.

Surgical treatment is planned on the basis of the amount of deviation, and the presence of associated horizontal deviations. In small deviations combined with horizontal deviation, a correction of the vertical element may be achieved by shifting the insertion of the horizontal muscle (5-8 mm) in the hypertropic eye, or shifting it up (to the same amount) in the hypotropic eye.

In large deviations, a recession of superior rectus of the hypertropic and recession of inferior oblique of the other eye is indicated.

DISSOCIATED VERTICAL DEVIATIONS (DVD)

It is basically a bilateral anomaly characterized by the hyperdeviation of either eye when the other eye is fixing. The hyperdeviation is accompanied by extortion and slight exodeviation. In this situation, if the fixing eye is covered, the squinting eye takes up fixation by moving down and in along with intortion. But, the covered eye does not make any movement, thus defying the Hering's law of ocular movements. That is why this type of vertical deviation is prefixed with the term 'Dissociated. It may be associated with any type of strabismus, any anomaly of binocular vision, nystagmus, or any defect ocular movements. On the other hand, it is seen as an isolated form. The etiology of this neuromuscular anomaly has not been explained clearly. Features—DVD is characterized by:

i. A spontaneous occurrence of vertical deviation of either eye when the patient is fatigued, or when fusion is interrupted by artificial means such as covering one eye.
ii. Lack of subjective symptoms in majority of case, an intermittent deviation being noticed by the onlookers—friends or parents. Some cases may have asthenopic symptoms. Diplopia is rare.
iii. Its frequent association with other forms of strabismus, specially with essential congenital exotropia and essential exotropia.
iv. Suppression in the nonfixing eye is present to eliminate diplopia.
v. Presence of peripheral fusion if there is no associated horizontal deviation.
vi. Presence of a facultative absolute scotoma, though bilateral, manifesting in the nonfixing eye.
vii. A frequent presence of latent nystagmus in cases of alternate DVD.

Diagnosis

The diagnosis of DVD is made on a careful assessment of the following tests.

Cover-Uncover Test

In a case of unilateral case of manifest DVD. When the fixing eye is covered, the deviating eye makes a downward movement unaccompanied by any downward movement of the uncovered eye.

- In a case of alternate DVD, either eye will show elevation under cover while the fixing eye will move down to take up fixation.
- In a case of a latent DVD, the eye under cover elevates but resumes fixation by making a downward movement. No movements take place in the uncovered eye.

Bielschowsky Phenomenon

It is usually present in cases of DVD. It is carried out by covering one eye, which deviates up under cover. While keeping the cover on, a photometric neutral filter wedge is placed in front of the fixing eye. As the filter wedge is placed before this eye it makes a downward movement which increases successively as the density of the filter is made to increase. Conversely, the deviating eye starts moving up successively as the density if the filter is made to decrease.

Treatment

i. Nonsurgical is of little value
ii. Surgical treatment is indicated when the condition presents a significant cosmetic problem. The following procedures have been recommended:
   a. *Recession of superior rectus*: A large recession (7-10 mm) may be done alone, or a small recession (3-5 mm) may be combined with anchoring of this muscle to the globe by nonabsorbable sutures, 12-15 mm behind its insertion (Faden operation).
   b. *Resection of inferior rectus*: This procedure may preferably be reserved for the cases showing a recurrence following large superior rectus recessions.
   c. *Combined operation*: This procedure has been recommended for large angle DVD particularly in rare cases which have a predominantly monocular vertical deviation with a hypertropia in primary position.

Recession of Inferior Oblique

This procedure which also includes anteriorisation of its insertion, is specially recommended for patients who have a DVD combined with an overaction of inferior oblique.

INCOMITANT VERTICAL DEVIATIONS

Various incomitant deviations caused by extraocular muscle palsies along with their sequelae had been dealt in the chapter on Paralytic Squints. However, there are two distinct entities which although cause incomitance, are different from other paralytic squints in many respects and can be discussed at this stage.

Inferior Oblique Overaction

It is characterized by an upshoot of the eye in adduction. The primary form is probably caused by some anatomical or innervational anomaly. It is seen either as an isolated anomaly or may be associated with esotropia or exotropia, oftenly having a V-pattern. The secondary form is caused by paresis of either its ipsilateral antagonist muscle (superior oblique), or its yoke muscle (contralateral superior rectus). The primary form has the following characteristics:

i. Onset is between 2-3 years of age
ii. It is frequently bilateral
iii. There is an upshoot or overelevation in the adducted position
iv. Horizontal squints are occasionally associated in the primary position
v. No head tilt is present
vi. Forced duction test is positive.

Treatment

The preferred surgical plan consists of a recession combined with antriorizaiton of inferior oblique muscle. In this procedure, the inferior muscle is detached from its insertion and reattached to the sclera near the lateral end of lateral rectus muscle. It is combined with the surgery if there is a concurrent horizontal squint.

Superior Oblique Overaction

It is characterized by a down shoot of the eye in adduction. The etiology is uncertain. Additional features are as follows:

i. It usually occurs by the age of 2-3 years
ii. It is frequently bilateral though may be asymmetrical at times
iii. It is commonly associated with concomitant esotropia or more commonly with exotropia
iv. Head tilt is absent
v. Forced duction test is positive.

Treatment

Treatment is indicated if there is a significant ocular deviation, or the presence of A-pattern. The recommended treatment consists of weakening of bilateral superior oblique muscles by way of tenotomy at the temporal or nasal border of superior rectus.

CYCLODEVIATIONS

Cyclodeviation (torsional strabismus) is of uncommon occurrence and refers to a misalignment of the eyes along the anteroposterior axis. Depending upon the direction of rotation, it may be classified as:

Excyclophoria or Excyclotropia

Excyclophoria or excyclotropia, when the 12 O'clock point on the cornea is rotated temporally.

Incyclophoria or Incyclotropia

Incyclophoria or incyclotropia, when the 12 O'clock point is turn nasally. This type of deviation is caused by an imbalance between the intorters (inferior oblique and superior rectus) and the extorters (superior oblique and inferior rectus) of the eyeball under the following situations:

i. Paresis or paralysis of a cyclovertical (particularly obliques) muscle
ii. Complication of surgical procedures on vertical or oblique muscles
iii. Manifestation of certain systemic diseases like Grave 1 disease, myasthenia gravis, etc.

A large majority of the patients are symptom-free. This is because of the development of suppression and anomalous retinal correspondence or on account of some physiological and psychological adaptations.

Treatment is indicated only in symptomatic patients and is always surgical.

13 A-V and X Syndromes

DEFINITION

The A and V syndrome consists of an abnormal variation in the amount of horizontal deviation as the eyes move from straight up to straight down positions of gaze or in other words "there is incomitency in the vertical positions of gaze." The shape of the letter 'A' symbolizes the increasing convergence down or increasing divergence up is symbolized by the letter 'V'.

CLASSIFICATION

Various classifications of the syndrome have been suggested from time to time. URIST (1951) suggested the following classification:

Group I

Esotropia with bilateral elevation in adduction. In these patients the esotropia is greater for near and in downward gaze than for distance and upward gaze, a right hypertropia on levoversion and a left hypertropia on dextroversion. The convergence to near point is good.

Group II

Esotropia with bilateral depression in adduction. In these patients the esotropia is greater for distance and in upward gaze than for near and in downward gaze a right hypertropia is present on to dextroversion and a left hypertropia on levoversion. The convergence to near point is good to fair.

Group III

Exotropia with bilateral elevation in adduction. In this group the exotropia is greater for distance and in upward gaze than for near and in downward gaze; right hypertropia is present on gaze to the left and a left hypertropia on gaze to the right. The convergence to near point is good.

Group IV

Exotropia with bilateral depression in adduction. In these patients the exotropia is greater for near and is downward gaze than for distance and upward gaze. A right hypertropia on gaze to the left. The convergence to near point is usually poor.

These syndrome has classified in a simple way, as follows:

1. V. esotropia—The esotropia is greater below than above.
2. A. esotropia—The esotropia is greater above than below.
3. V. exotropia—The exotropia is greater above than below.
4. A. exotropia—The exotropia is greater below than above.

Thus, he gave the name of 'A' and 'V' syndrome to vertically incomitant squint and described A and V esotropia and exotropia. He did not define the limits of normal deviation in the up and down position of gaze. There is a new classification to rectify the previous deficiencies and included even those cases which would otherwise not fit in.

Pure Type

There is a variation in the horizontal strabismus as the patient looks up and down with nonvertical incomitance in any of the nine position of gaze. This may be further divided into 'A' or 'V' type of esotropia or exotropia.

Impure Type

Besides the horizontal strabismus which occurs on looking up and down, there is vertical incomitance in one or more of the other positions of gaze. This group may be further subdivided into 3 patterns.

i. The left eye remains hypertropic on dextroversion and right eye on levoversion.
ii. The right eye remains hypertropic on dextroversion and left eye on levoversion.
iii. The same eye hypertropic on both dextro and levoversion.

INCIDENCE

There has been no exact agreement on the frequency of occurrence of the 'A' and 'V' pattern in strabismus. Various authors have given varying incidence as shown in the Table 13.1.

TABLE 13.1: Incidence of A-V pattern in strabismus

S. No.	*Author and year*	*Incidence*
1.	Urist 1951	50%
2.	Knapp. 1959	12.5%

CLINICAL PICTURE

The clinical characteristics of patients with A and V pattern shall now be considered.

1. V – esotropia – Following features characterize this condition.
   a. Eso greater below (V)
   b. May be overaction of oblique, inferior rectus, medial rectus

   If there is an abnormal head position, the chin is depressed to bring the eyes upwards for this is the most favorable position possible to minimize the deviation. Another clinical characteristic which is occasionally observed is the clumsiness of three patients in going downstairs.
2. A – esotropia. This is characterized by:
   a. Eso greater above than below
   b. May be over action of superior rectus or superior oblique
   c. May be underaction of inferior rectus or inferior oblique.

   Patient with A exotropia tend to assume the chin up and binocular vision in this particular direction of gaze.
3. V – exotropia. This is characterized by:
   a. Exo greater above
   b. May be over action of inferior oblique
   c. May be under action superior rectus or superior oblique.

   This group comprises those patients who had greater exotropia – constant or intermittent – in upward gaze. If there is an abnormal head position, it will be a chin up and eyes down position.
4. A – exotropia is characterized by:
   a. Exo greater below (A)
   b. May be over action of superior oblique or superior rectus
   c. May be under action of inferior oblique or inferior rectus.

A chin down and eyes up posture may be assumed by same and this may lead to clumsiness going downstairs.

ETIOLOGY

The exact etiology of this syndrome is still controversial. Various factors are considered to underline this mechanism of A and V syndromes.

Anatomical Factors

Although anatomical anomalies do not cause A:V syndrome in all cases, there are a number of clinical entities which create true 'A' and 'V' patterns. This in the superior oblique tend on sheath syndrome of Brown it is common to encounter a V pattern. This is attributed to the action of the incelastic superior oblique sheath as a grey line forcing divergence in elevation. The adherence syndrome (adherence of lateral rectus with inferior oblique or superior rectus with superior oblique) may create a mechanical vergence shift in the vertical fields.

Of considerable interest, although lacking explanation are the patterns associated with anomalies of the palpebral fissures and facial bones first pointed out by Urist. There is association of the 'V' pattern and overaction of inferior oblique in patients with mongoloid palpebral fissures.

Innervational Factors

Horizontal Muscle School

Horizontal recti Urist (1951) is believer of this school and the thinks that A and V syndrome can result from dysfunction of the horizontal rectus muscles. He feels that basically there is exaggeration of the normal tendency of exodeviation to increase in upward gazes and of esodeviation to increase in downward gaze. Thus, a defect greater in upward gaze is said to be due to lateral rectus dysfunction; V – exotropia representing overaction of lateral rectus and 'A' exotropia representing under action of medial rectus muscle. The following arguments support this theory that A and V syndrome are produced by the dysfunction of the horizontal muscles.

i. Correction of the different angle of strabismus that exists in the upward and downward gazes through proper surgical treatment of the affected horizontal muscles.
ii. Uneven results in the straight up and straight down position of gaze as a result of the operation mistakenly performed on unaffected horizontal muscles.

   Urist showed in a case, the effects of incorrect surgical treatment consisting of 4 mm recession of both medial recti in 'A' esotropia that led to an exotropia of 5-10° in looking up and 20° on looking down. He suggested that proper surgery in this case for A esotropia would have been the resection of both lateral recti.

iii. Elimination of vertical deviation after operations on horizontal muscles only.

iv. Replacement of one syndrome by another with conversion of the apparent under action of the vertical muscle into opposite defect after an operation on horizontal muscle. Resection of both lateral recti and recession of medial recti changed the clinical picture into V – esotropia with moderate spasm of both inferior oblique. It is noteworthy that by an operation on horizontal muscle only and with the passage of time the apparent paralysis of both inferior oblique were changed into spasm. This supports that the A – esotropia was of secondary nature.

v. A and V syndrome without abnormalities in the action of vertical muscle.

Vertical Muscle School

There is another school of thought which believes that the syndrome is the result of a primary defect in vertical muscles. The opinions however, divided: one group believing the obliques to be it fault while the other group believing the defect in vertical rectus to be responsible. This abnormality may be manifested through the secondary function of adduction and abduction of the obliques and vertical recti respective.

Oblique muscle defect: This group feels that in defects greater in the upward gaze, the inferior obliques are at fault. Thus, V—exotropia would be due to overacting inferior obliques and A—esotropia due to underacting inferior since the obliques assessory abductors.

Defects greater in the downward gaze are attributed to superior oblique dysfunction. Thus A exotropia is due to overacting superior oblique and V – esotropia due to underacting superior oblique. Jamplosky (1957) is an exponent of this school.

Rectus muscles: This group feels that when defect is greater in the upward gaze, the superior recti are at fault. Thus V-exo would be due to underacting superior recti since superior recti are assessory adductors. Similarly, defects greater in downward are attributed to inferior recti dysfunction. Thus, A—exotropia would be due to underacting inferior recti and veso would be due to overacting inferior recti.

Combined School

There is yet another school which has varied ideas regarding etiology. Accordingly it is felt that the horizontal recti may be at fault in some instances and the vertical acting muscles in other or there may be combined dysfunction of both the group of muscles. It is logical since the vertical defects appear in gazes where both sets of vertically acting muscles are working in combination with horizontal muscles or in other words a form of synergic dysfunction exists. Some of the authors have put forward the following clinical arguments in favor of the idea that the bilateral vertical deviation are primary and not secondary in A and V syndrome.

a. Cases of A and V syndrome without horizontal strabismus in primary position.
b. Cases in which vertical deviation persists after the horizontal muscle have been operated upon and second operation on the vertical muscles was needed to correct the vertical deviation.

It is possible to come across A and V syndrome without horizontal strabismus but such cases are very rare. Great majority of cases with A and V syndrome manifest either as convergent. Dysfunction of the medial recti and atrophy of the lateral recti. There may be an interventional oberration whereby the horizontal recti are functional connected to the vertical muscles V tropies the medial recti may be related to the oblique and the lateral rectus muscle may be similarly related vertical rectus muscle.

Gobin (1968) felt that the cause of 'V' phenomenon may be due to change in the angle between visual existence muscle axis. For example, He presumes that the 'A' incomitance is due to a torsional imbalance between the two oblique muscles. This due to a reduction of the angle between the superior oblique and visual axis. This is termed a sagittalization of the muscles; it increases the vertical and reduces the torsional action, adding to excyclophoria. This excyclophoria can be compensated by a contraction of the intorsional muscles and an inhibition the extorsional muscles, i.e. a contraction of the superior rectus and superior oblique and inhibition of the inferior rectus and inferior oblique. This change in contraction of the vertical muscle produces a depression in adduction and an 'A' variation of the horizontal angle of squint.

The 'V' incomitance is also due to lack of torsional balance between the obliques, caused in this case by a legitimization of the inferior oblique.

The angle between his muscle and the visual axis is reduced, and this results in a decreased extorsional and an increased vertical action leading to encyclophoria. This encyclophoria of the eyes can be compensated for by a contraction of the extorsional muscles and an inhibition of the intorsional muscles, i.e. a contraction of the inferior rectus and inferior oblique and inhibition of the superior rectus and superior oblique.

X-incomitance is due to a torsional imbalance between the oblique on the one hand and the vertical rectus on the other. This may be due to a sagittalization of both the oblique, whereby their torsional action is decreased and there up and excyclophoria on looking down. On looking up the extorsional muscles will be contracted and the intorsional muscles will be contracted and the extorsional muscles inhibited, i.e. on elevation there is contraction of the inferior oblique and inhibition of the superior rectus and on depression there is contraction of the superior oblique and inhibition of the inferior rectus.

DIAGNOSIS

Electromyographic Studies

In V type exotropias the electrical activity of lateral recti increased and that of medial recti reciprocally inhibited in upward gaze. In A type exotropias the identical changes occurred in downward gaze. Corresponding alternations appear in A and V exotropias. He therefore concluded that the horizontal recti must play part in the varying angle of strabismus.

The more presence of increased activity of muscle may on by reflect the new position of eye rather than tell us why the eye moved to this position. For example, if the eye of an exophore is covered that eye will deviate under cover and the electromyogram will show increased activity of the lateral rectus of that eye. This does not mean that an abnormally overactive lateral rectus caused exophoria. It simply means that eyes are moved by the eye muscle and that in this case the deviated eye was pulled outwards by its lateral rectus muscle.

Electromyographically at the deviating eye experiences innovational shift in both vertical and horizontal muscle as it moves into the oblique position. This shift of horizontal innovation is not seen in the fixating eye which simple rotates in a vertical meridian. He therefore concluded that the horizontal muscles also exert an influence upon the pattern and these patterns are influenced my both vertical as well as horizontal muscle.

Method of Testing

1. A vertical imbalance should be noted whether or not it is bilaterally is symmetrical equal and in accordance with the theoretical pattern. Facial bony pattern and shape should be noted as.
2. Full refractive correction should done because uncorrected ametropia may produce variable findings.
3. It is important to control accommodation by having the patient fixate a small letter or picture to eliminate accommodation with plus 3.00 D sphere for near measurements an 'A' and 'V' pattern may be stimulated by difference in accommodation convergency in various direction of gaze.
4. Although demonstration of the 'A' and 'V' pattern for distance and near is sufficient to make the diagnosis but for sake of completeness, midline measurement in up gaze and down gaze be made for both distance and near. More accurate would be to use synaptophore for the measurement at 25° upward gaze and 25° of downward gaze to demonstrate. A and V pattern which may be misused just by measuring the angle for squint by Hirschberg's method.

In order to diagnose a clinically 'V' pattern there much be a difference of 15 prism diopters between up gaze and down gaze. Similarly in order to make a diagnosis of a clinically significant 'A' pattern there must be a 10 diopter difference between up gaze and down gaze.

It has been known that eyes tend to diverge in upward gaze and to coverage in downward gaze. The fact that we ordinarily look up in distance vision and look down in near vision has been given importance in this phenomenon.

Because of this mild built in V-pattern the above limit for A and V have been suggested.

Difference in the Pattern

Neither all patients with an 'A' and 'V' pattern have a demonstrable vertical dysfunction nor do all patients with vertical dysfunction display an 'A' and 'V' pattern. For example, we have V-esotropias with overaction of the inferior oblique, V esotropia with no discernible muscle dysfunction and V esotropia with under action of the inferior oblique.

Although these are V–esotropias they manifest in or different fashion and the survival approach that would cure one type may be quite disappointing in the others.

Importance of Version

Versions are of special importance in the diagnosis of 'A' and 'V' pattern overaction and underactions of vertical muscles require more consideration here than in tropias which are horizontally comitant in vertical gaze.

Tests for Fusion

It should be done on all cases. It is important to discover whether there is single binocular vision present and in what field of gaze. Obviously, fusion should be preserved it possible for the sake of future stability. Everyone is concerned with how the eyes look, we must be equally concerned with how the eyes see.

Role of Orthoptic Examination

A detailed orthoptic examination in all such cases is essential for proper diagnosis and aid in management. Lee'sor Hess screening whenever possible should always be done to find associated condition of various muscles in an attempt to find the etiological factor which may have a bearing the treatment.

TREATMENT

It is surgical and only surgical. There are no nonsurgical means by which these conditions can be influenced directly. It should be apparent that there is a variety of approaches to the surgical treatment of the 'A' and 'V' pattern.

I. The most commonly performed operations for strabismus are recession or resection operations on the horizontal muscle which might influence the A and V pattern.
II. While doing so their insertions may be transplanted upward or downwards thus changing the mechanical advantage of muscles which might influence the A and V pattern.
III. Since vertical recti are secondary adductors weakening or straightening of their action might increase or decrease their adducting effect thus influencing the A or V pattern.
IV. To modify the adducting affect of vertical recti their insertions. May be moved usually to enhance adduction or temporarily to diminish adduction.
V. The oblique muscles are secondary abductions. Their weakening should, therefore reduce abduction and their strengthen enhance abduction.

These approaches do not always produce the expected results as extraocular muscles act in pairs and groups and so operation on an muscle influences the other. For these reasons the applicability of these approaches must be treated against actual experience with various surgical procedures.

Horizontal Recti

The lateral rectus are attacked if the defect is greater upward. Thus in V-exodeviation there will be weakened while in A eso they would be strengthened. If the defect is greatest below the medial recti are attacked in an identical manner, i.e. in V-esodeviation they would be weakened while in A-exodeviation they would be strengthened.

With these there is a definite risk of over correction in the field of least deviation if the field of greatest deviation is fully corrected — a 'V' esodeviation can at times be converted into a V-exodeviation.

In an effort to minimize this, supra or infraplacement of the horizontal muscles insertion is tried. These are done in an effort to alter the function more in one vertical position than in other. There is some disagreement as to the direction in which placement should be done. One group infraplaces the medial recti to obtain increased action in upward gaze. While the other group will supraplace these for a similar purpose.

The horizontal recti should be placed in the direction if increased function is the aim. For example, in V- eso the medial recti will be recorded and placed downwards in an effort to lessen more adduction in the downward gaze where as in A – exo the medial recti will be resected and supraplaced in an effort to achieve increased adduction in the lower gaze as compared to upward gaze. The amount of displacement may vary from a few mm to a full width of tendon, on the severity of the vertical incomitance and individual surgeons choice. This type of surgery is suitable for cases in which there are no vertically overaction or underacting muscles.

Vertical Muscle School

As we know whenever there is an over action of inferior oblique, there is 'V' pattern both is eso and exotropia. Weakening of inferior oblique is therefore the operation of choice. This would reduce the 'V' pattern by increasing an esotropia in the upper field of fixation and by decreasing an exotropia in the same field. A paradical effect, i.e. a reduction in the esotropia or an increase in the exotropia may sometimes be seen.

Occasionally, the combined efforts in the upper or lower field may be so great as to charge V esodeviation or V exodeviation into A eso or A exodeviation.

In A esodeviation inferior oblique would be a strength by resecting and advancing them. The superior oblique are utilized if the defect is greatest in the downward gaze. Thus in A exodeviation they would be weakened and in V – esodeviation they would be strengthened.

Vertical Recti

This school utilized the secondary function of adduction of the vertical recti as the basis of their surgical approach. Superior recti are attacked when the imbalance is greatest in upward gaze. Thus in V – exodeviation the superior recti would be strengthened and in an A – eso they would be weakened.

A second maneuver is available here as compared to supra- and infraplacement of the horizontal recti. It consists of nasal placement of vertical recti insertions when increased adduction is required and temporal placement when decreased adduction is aimed at. There is no controversy regarding this as in horizontal recti. The amount of placement may vary. The average is about 5 to 7 mm. In extreme cases the muscle could be moved midway between its formal insertion and the horizontal rectus insertion. This may be combined with a resection or recession depending upon the severity of the defect and the opinion of the individual surgeon. The resection and recession should be done with great caution here.

Combined School

Since according to this group either the horizontal or vertical recti are at fault, so the surgical approach also varies. When there is no vertical muscle component, they follow the techniques of horizontal recti school usually doing a weakening or strengthening procedure combined with supra- or infraplacements. If there is a demonstrable symmetrical vertical defect, they attack either of the vertical muscles. But there is a unilateral or asymmetrical vertical defect or one does not fit into theoretical pattern, this vertical component will be handled by standard vertical surgery.

In addition to the A and V patterns, some other pattern have also been described.

1. X- phenomenon. This consist of two components.
   a. *Horizontal incomitance*: The angle of deviation is more convergent in the primary position than on looking up or down.

b. *Vertical incomitance*: In looking up there is elevation in adduction and looking up there is elevation in adduction and looking down there is depression in adduction. In symmetrical X phenomenon the incomitance is equal in elevation and depression. In the asymmetrical types the relative divergence is less on looking up than is looking down. (XA–phenomenon) or the relative divergence is great on looking up than on looking down (XV–phenomenon).

2. Y–phenomenon–In this case the eyes are orthophoric in primary position and in downward gaze but show an increased divergence in upward gaze. The reverse phenomenon and have called it an inverted Y–pattern.

14 Musculofascial Anomalies

There are a group of certain congenital disorder of ocular motility in which the pathology is usually in the musculofascial system of the orbital. These anomalies have certain feature in common.

CLINICAL FEATURES

1. Gross limitation of ocular movements in one or more direction of gaze with small angle of deviation with orthophoria in the primary position.
2. Some limitation of ocular movement observed in the direction opposite to that of the main limitation.
3. Some retraction of the affected eyeball and narrowing of palpebral fissure when the eye is rotated in a certain direction usually opposite to that of main limitation of movement and there is some widening of palpebral fissure in the direction of main limitation of movement.
4. Forced duction test is positive. But if the primary affected muscle is one of the recti then the rigidity of the affected muscle cannot be tested by forced duction test.

FORCED DUCTION TEST

Indications

To assess the degree of a paresis of muscle or the presence of a contracture, fibrosis or incarceration. This can be done by possible degrees of rotation of the globe by various methods.

Forced Duction Test of Goldstein

Through the anesthetized conjunctiva near the limbus, the tendon of the muscle is grasped by toothed forceps while another forceps grasps the belly of offending muscle. If the forceps cannot be made to approach one another easily then there is rigidity of this muscle or its sheath or it is incarcerated. Then forced duction test is positive.

Forced Duction Test of Scott

The conjunctiva near the limbus over the attachment of the paretic muscle is held by nontoothed forceps and while it is held steadily, an attempt is made to move the eye in field of action of the muscle so that it power can be assessed. The eye can also be moved away from the field of action of the muscle in a simple paresis. There is a full excursion of the globe in this direction, but this is limited in the presence of abnormal rigidity of the muscle or its sheath.

DIVISION

Pathology of congenital musculofascial anomalies can be divided as follows:

Congenital Anomalies in the Insertions or Tendons of Muscles

Fibrosis of the Muscles

Congenital anomalies in the insertions or tendons of muscles.

1. Absence or hypoplasia of muscles: Most common: inferior rectus
2. Fusion of muscles: Due to
   i. Defective cleavage in developing mesoderm
   ii. Fusion of tendons fusion of fascial sheath, e.g. Adherence syndrome
3. Fibrous bands
4. Abnormal insertions.

Commonest Cause of Congenital Defects in Ocular Motility

Fascial anomalies: Resulting from thickening of intermuscular membrane and the incorporation of latter into muscular fibre resulting in obstruction to adequate contraction and relaxation.

FIBROTIC RETRACTION OF MUSCLE

Duane's Retraction Syndrome

This was initially described by Stilling (1887) and Turk (1896). Hence also known as Stilling–Turk-Duane's syndrome. This is most common type of musculofascial anomaly seen more commonly in females.

Etiology

Myogenic factors

1. Producing retraction
   a. Posterior insertion of medial rectus
   b. Presence of a flat, broad, tendinous band attaché behind the insertion of medial rectus
   c. Fixation of the globe by a fibrotic lateral rectus muscle.
2. Producing narrowing of palpebral aperture
   a. Ptosis as a passive process secondary to retraction of the globe.
3. Producing vertical movements
   a. Oblique muscle overaction to compensate for an ineffective lateral rectus muscle
   b. Overaction of vertical recti to compensate for the ineffective medial rectus
   c. Cocontraction of horizontal recti augmenting their vertical action
   d. Resistance offered by optic nerve in the direction of retraction causing a vertical movement of the globe.

Neurogenic factors

1. Electromyography reveals absence of electrical activity in lateral rectus muscle on attempted abduction. This paradoxical behavior of lateral rectus could be due to innervation of the muscle by IIIrd nerve instead of VIth nerve.
2. Cocontraction of the horizontal recti could be cause of retraction of the globe.
3. Abnormal synergistic action between the medial rectus and superior and inferior recti or oblique muscles have also been found electromyographically which may explain the vertical movements in some cases.
4. At present it is believed that Duane's retraction syndrome is an innervation disturbance of muscular or supranuclear origin rather than a structural anomaly.

Acquired Duane's Retraction Syndrome

It has been reported following head injury or with brainstem tumor. Iatrogenic Duane's syndrome following removal of dermolipoma has also been reported.

Inverse Duane's Retraction Syndrome

Characterized by restriction of adduction and retraction on abduction Degeneration of medial rectus muscle in medial orbital has been implicated as its cause.

Type I: Most common
Characterized by:
1. Marked restriction or total absence of abduction
2. Normal or mildly restricted adduction
3. In the primary position, straight or slightly esotropic eyes
4. Narrowing of palpebral aperture with some degree of ptosis on adduction
5. On abduction, there is widening of palpebral aperture.

Type II: Characterized by:
1. Limitation of adduction and there is retraction on attempted adduction
2. Normal or mildly limited abduction
3. Eyes may be orthophoric or there may be esophoria/esotropia.

Type III: Characterized by:
1. Gross restriction of adduction
2. Slight limitation of abduction
3. Retraction on attempted adduction.

Patients with Duane's syndrome are orthophoric in primary position or they may be adopt a suitable head posture to enjoy uniocular single vision. There may be upshoot or down shoot of the eye in adduction.

Associated Congenital Anomaly

1. Perceptive deafness with associated speech disorder
2. Iris stroma dysplasia
3. Pupillary abnormalities
4. Cataract
5. Persistent hyaloid arteries
6. Choroidal colobomas
7. Crocodile tears
8. Goldenhar's syndrome
9. Klippel-Feil anomaly
10. Cervical spina bifida
11. Labyrinthine deafness

Duane's syndrome associated with deafness and Klippel-Feil anomaly constitute.

Wildervanck's Syndrome

Treatment

No treatment.

a. When eyes are straight in primary position
b. No amblyopia.

Indications for surgery

a. Cosmetic—abnormal head posture
b. Manifest squint interfering with binocular functions.

Surgery

A. *When esotropia is present:* Recession of the medial rectus of affected eye accompanied by a free tenotomy of any abnormal bands.

Recession of the medial rectus of normal eye may be necessary as a secondary procedure.

B. *When exotropia is present:* Ipsilateral lateral rectus recession with contralateral medial rectus resection can be done. Lateral rectus resection must never be done as it has little effect on the angle of deviation and it further aggravate retraction. Recession of lateral rectus has a beneficial effect on retraction with no worsening of abduction weakness.

Surgeries intended to reduce the esodeviation usually aggravate adduction weakness.

C. Posterior fixation suture of the contralateral medial rectus or ipsilateral lateral rectus (**Faden procedure**) has also been advocated.

Disadvantage of Surgery

Full range of ocular movement can never be achieved.

Vertical Retraction Syndrome

- Rare congenital condition
- Vertical recti are involved.

Characterized by limitation of movement of affected eye on elevation or depression associated with retraction of globe and narrowing of palpebral fissure.

The affected eye thus shows hypotropia on looking upwards and outwards and hypertropia on looking downwards and outwards while orthophoria may be only be evident on depression.

Forced duction test indicates that the lesion is due to the restriction of movement of the affected muscle itself.

Superior Oblique Sheath Syndrome of Brown

First described in 1950's by Brown.

Etiology

1. Here the sheath of the superior oblique tendon is congenitally shortened. Forced duction test becomes dramatically negative following stripping of the sheath. Some evidence have shown fibrous connections between tendon and sheath.
2. Thickening of tendon sheath has also been noticed, e.g. unusual manifestation of rheumatoid arthritis.
3. *Tendon anomalies*: Cases have been reported in whom repeated attempt to elevate the adducted eye result in a sudden release of resistance. The eye regains full motility. There are cases in whom intermittent Brown's syndromes is present which disappears with a click—superior oblique click syndrome. All these cases points towards some kind of resistance in the path of the tendon.
4. *Anomalies of inferior oblique muscle*: Anomalies of sheath of inferior oblique muscle have been implicated. Case report of fibrous bands between inferior oblique and lateral wall are available. Also cases of Brown's syndrome following blow out fracture of the orbital floor has been reported.
5. Paradoxical innervation of the superior oblique muscle has been hypothesized by some authors, who belived that superior oblique loses its ability to relax and subsequently goes into contracture.

Acquired Brown's Syndrome

It has been reported following:

1. Blunt injury to the eye
2. Following superior oblique tucking procedure (strengthening procedure)
3. Secondary to inferior oblique palsy

Clinical Features

1. Usually found in children
2. More often unilateral and usually sporadic
3. Shows dominant tendency when inherited
4. Eyes usually straight or hypotropic in primary position
5. Limited right elevation in adduction
6. Normal right elevation in abduction
7. No or minimal superior oblique overaction
8. Positive forced duction test on elevating the globe on adduction
9. Down shoot in adduction
10. Anomalous head position with idiopathic head tilt and chin up to opposite side to compensate for some excyclotropia.

Differential Diagnosis

1. *Inferior oblique palsy*: Forced duction test is negative, i.e. there is no resistance to elevation in adduction. Also there is no depression on adduction, normal action of ipsilateral superior oblique and contralateral superior rectus and there is no V-phenomena.
2. *Orbital floor fracture*: There is restriction of elevation not only in adduction, but also in direct elevation.

Treatment

Treatment of Brown's syndrome yields unsatisfactory results. Spontaneous recovery is known in acquired cases.

Indication for Surgery

1. Presence of primary position hypotropia and an anomalous head posture
2. When torticollis becomes a cosmetic problem.

Procedure

Dissection and stripping of tendon sheath is a logical solution.

Superior Oblique Tenotomy

Many result in symptoms of palsy necessitating secondary surgery usually inferior oblique recession of the same side or inferior rectus recession again on the same side.

Strabismus Fixus

In this congenital anomaly, one or both the eyes are fixed in either the convergent position caused by fibrous tightening of the medial recti (convergent strabismus fixus) or fibrosis of lateral recti (divergent strabismus fixus).

No horizontal movement is possible. Patient developed a variable head posture. There is no diplopia, suppression is frequent, usually no amblyopia as the patient tends to use both eyes alternately. Binocular functions are poor.

Divergent strabismus fixus and vertical strabismus fixus are rare.

Treatment

Liberal recession of medial recti along with recession of conjunctiva and Tenon's capsule. Abduction beyond midline can never be achieved. As a general rule the patient compensates for the loss of movements of the eye with free rotation of this head.

Fibrosis of the Extraocular Muscles

Rare familial disorder involving most or all extraocular muscles.

Clinical Features

1. Downwards fixation of both eyes
2. Severe ptosis
3. Perverted convergence on attempted elevation or on looking to the side.

   Inheritance is autosomal dominant.

Differential Diagnosis

1. Blow out fracture of the orbital floor.
2. Brown's syndrome
3. Double elevator palsy
4. Endocrine myopathy

Treatment

By complete inferior rectus tenotomy. Ptosis surgery may be done.

Adherence Syndrome

Sheaths of lateral rectus and inferior oblique muscles may be adherent causing pseudoparalysis of lateral rectus. Adhesions between superior rectus and superior oblique may present with pseudoparalysis of superior rectus.

Treatment

By lysis of these adhesions.

15 Abnormal Retinal Correspondence

Normal retinal correspondence is said to exist in a person when retinal elements in the two eyes (for example, the two foveae) which should have a common visual direction, activity prove to possess it. Normal retinal correspondence is the most fundamental fact in binocular vision. It is based on the anatomic and physiologic organization of the organ of vision, it is not acquired in the course of individual development.

On the other hand abnormal retinal correspondence (ARC) is the rearrangement of the common visual direction of retinal elements of the two eyes, corresponding retinal elements loosing then common visual direction and is said to exist when the fovea of one eye is used simultaneously with a retinal area other than fovea of the squinting eye. It is a functional sensory adaptation consequent to strabismus to avoid diplopia and confusion and to restore some form of binocular vision. This adaptation is brought about by an inherent desire for some form of binocular vision and to avoid diplopia and confusion that would otherwise take place. It is due to an interpretation or adaptation at a cortical level abnormal retinal correspondence is a binocular condition. In the presence of ocular deviation with normal retinal correspondence with binocular function diplopia results, as the protection is correct to the altered position of the eye. But in abnormal retinal correspondence, in spite of the ocular deviation the projection is straight ahead and no diplopia results. Objective localization in the space does not coincide with the subjective localization, while dealing with a care of abnormal retinal correspondence, in every subjective test the projection is correct in spite of the deviation and there are constant discrepancies between the objective and subjective visual space. Abnormal retinal correspondence was first coined by Chavsse in 1939. The other term used for it are anomalous correspondence, anomalous projection and anomalous binocular function. ARC may be harmonious or unharmonious. It is said to be harmonious when the angle of anomaly is equal to the angle of deviation and unharmonious when the angle of anomaly is less than the angle of the squint. *Harmonious Abnormal Retinal Correspondence,* this is a type of abnormal retinal correspondence in which the area of the retina of the squinting eye stimulated by an object, during the fixation of that object by the fovea of the nonsquinting eye, assumes an abnormal type of projection, so that image of the object is appreciated in a straight head direction. *Unharmonious Anomalous Retinal Correspondence,* this is a type of abnormal retinal correspondence in which the area of the retina of squinting eye stimulated by an object, during fixation of that object. By fovea of the nonsquinting eye, assumes an abnormal type of projection, so that image of the object is appreciated to the side of the fixation object in a direction opposite to that of the direction of the squint. Incidence of ARC varies quiet significantly depending upon the method of assessment. It varies from 0.6 to 92%, which in itself betrays any agreement on it incidence.

DEVELOPMENT OF ABNORMAL RETINAL CORRESPONDENCE

There have been various views on the development of ARC various theories put forward by different people. According to empirical theory retinal correspondence was acquired and not congenital and that we learn the relationship of the retinal points to each other by means of eye movement, and that macular correspondence is formed by the correlation of sight and touch, the two macula'e being the most sensitive points of vision and therefore directed towards the object we use to notice. The more often we repeat this process the more fixed is the relationship of the retinal. The visual directions determined by the spatial value of the retinal elements are not fixed in space absolutely. They change with the position of the eyes and are only fixed relative in the visual direction of the fovea. Which is termed the principle visual direction. In normal retinal correspondence the fovea of the fixating eye and the extramacular element of the deviated eye have common visual direction. It implies that here is single vision with there two, originally disperate retinal elements. It is apparent therefore that abnormal retinal correspondence represents an adaptation of the sensory apparatus of the eyes to the abnormal position of the eyes. According to another theory innate theory for development of ARC is based on this assumption that local sign of each retinal element and the type of retinal correspondence are present since birth. There is some connection between each retinal area with the cortical area and corresponding retinal elements in each retina have connection with the same cortical area, and fusion is due to the excitation of single cortical area by the two separate corresponding retinal elements with this hypothesis the phenomenon of stereopsis cannot be explained because stereopsis or depth perception is perceived by stimulation of disparate retinal elements.

Harmonious anomalous correspondence is said to exist as the shift in visual directions to such an extent that it has completely effect the angle of squint. It the shift in visual direction is less extensive than would be required by the duration then unharmonious anomalous correspondence is said to exist. In the development of an anomalous correspondence the angle of anomaly gradually increases until it finally reaches and amount equal to that of the angle of squint. Before this final stage of harmonious correspondence, the stage of unharmonious correspondence was developing. All cases of abnormal retinal correspondence has harmonious relationship to start with and the unharmonious state develops because of slight change in the angle of squint. The concept of gradual attempts by the patients to achieve a harmonious type of ARC as a result of the progressive and purposive change in the degree of unharmonious element is widely accepted.

Relationship of ARC with the Age of Onset of the Squint

Anomalous correspondence is found more commonly in persons in whom the deviation of the visual axes arose early in life ARC is more prevalent when the onset of squint is before 4years of age as compared to after this age. This anomalous, adaptation requires individual adoptability as well as time for it to become deeply rooted. The younger the patient is at the time of onset of squint, the more readily and more speedily it develops.

Relationship of ARC with the Type of Squint

ARC is more common in esotropia than in exotropia. Anomalous correspondence is for more prevalent in the alternating type.

In paralytic squints the sensory adaptation are rare. It may be present only in those cases where the paralysis has occurred in the very early childhood or is congenital and a long duration of time has elapsed or they have developed a secondary concomitance. In microtropia anomalous correspondence is a rule and is a primary and hereditary defect.

Relationship of ARC with Angle of Squint

With very small angle, ARC is the rule. Harmonious anomalous correspondence prevails in patients with low degree of strabismus 30 or less whereas suppression is the rule in larger duration.

Relationship of ARC with Suppression and Amblyopia

Anomalous correspondence and suppression coexist in patients with concomitant strabismus. Harmonious ARC prevails in patients of low degree of squint, while suppression is the rule in duration larger than 30°.

DIAGNOSIS OF ABNORMAL RETINAL CORRESPONDENCE

Well-established abnormal retinal correspondence is a serious obstacle to the recovery of the normal binocular vision and preexisting abnormal retinal correspondence also influence the postoperative results so it is very important to diagnose the state of retinal correspondence. For this purpose, various tests are listed in Table 15.1.

TABLE 15.1: Ovarian tests for ARC

- Synoptophore test
- The after image test
- Bagolini's striated glasses test
- Worth Fur-dot test
- Bifoveal correspondence test
- Projected after image test
- Maddox wing test
- Maddox rod test
- Diplopia test
- Double image test
- Mirror screen test
- Phase difference haploscopy
- Projection or polorized test
- Hallden test
- Vertical prism test of Fitton
- The screen test
- The congruouce test of Tschermak.

Synoptophore Test

The patient was seated before the synoptophore and the instrument adjusted according to the patient's height and interpupillary distance. Depending upon the patient's visual acuity, foveal, parafoveal, macular or paramacular slides were used. First the objective angle was measured by flashing the tubes alternately and observing for any movement of either eye. The tubes were manipulated in a way that movement of eyes was eliminated on alternate flashing. The objective angle was read on the scale when the objective angle was measured patient was asked to put the lion into the cage. The angle at which the patient was able to put the lion into the cage was taken as the subjective angle and the difference between the two was angle of anomaly.

If the subjective angle was equal to the angle measured objectively than the cases were said to have normal retinal correspondence. Then the angle of anomaly (i.e. the difference between the subjective and the objective angle) was equal to the objective. Angle, they were said to have harmonious abnormal retinal correspondence. If on the other hand, the angle of anomaly was less than the objective angle but more than zero, then the cases were supposed to have unharmonious abnormal retinal correspondence. The cases who were able to see the two slide simultaneously but could not put the lion into the cage, then the angle of crossing was taken as the subjective angle.

Bagolini's Striated Glasses Test

First the angle of the squint was measured by the prism bar cover test. Then the patient was asked to fix a spotlight at a distance of 30 cm and then at a distance of 6 meters as the case may be after asking the patient to wear the trial frame, Bagolini's striated glasses were put on before each eye. The glasses were put in a manner so that striations of the glass in front of one eye was at right angle to the striations of the glass in the other eye. If a patient with a manifest squint saw a spotlight crossed in the center by two lines, the patient was supposed to have harmonious abnormal retinal correspondence. If he saw two spots, each intersected by a separate line then appropriate prisms, base in or base out in exotropes and esotropes respectively, were placed in front of one eye till the patient started seeing one spotlight with two lines crossing at right angle to each other. The strength of the prism required to produce this effect was noted. If the strength of the prism was equal to the object angle of the squint then patient was supposed to have normal retinal correspondence. If the strength of the prism was less than the objective angle then the presence of unharmonious abnormal retinal correspondence was declared suppression of one eye was indicated when patient could appreciated only one spotlight with one line crossing it at a time.

After-Image Test

This test was conducted on major amblyoscopes. The test was carried out in a semi-darkroom. The tubes were set at zero opal filters were removed and the specially designed slides, one with a horizontal slit, another with a vertical slit and each having a red spot in the center for fixation, were inserted in the slide slot. Now each eye was stimulated in turn for twenty seconds (to eliminate the suppressions) eye and this eye was stimulated in the end, i.e. after the nonsuppressing eye was simulated. During the flashing patient was instructed to fix at the central red spot on the slide and not to move the eyes. Simultaneously a watch was kept on the patient's eyes. After each eye was flashed, opal filters were reinserted slides were removed and binocular flashing device was switched as to facilitate the after image. Now patient was told to look at the illuminated white screen and was asked to draw that he sees. If patient was as complete cross is indicated that patient has normal retinal correspondence. If the patient sees the incomplete cross. Then the patient was declared to be having abnormal retinal correspondence. If the patient sees only one line it indicated that patient has suppression of the other eye.

A. Normal localization in NRC
B. Abnormal localization in esotropes
C. Abnormal localization in exotropes.

Worth's Four Dot Test

Four dot test can be utilized for diagnosing the state of retinal correspondence. If the patient sees four dots in presence of manifest squint if indicates abnormal retinal correspondence. The patient wears red glass before the right eye and green glass before the left eye. At a distance of 6 meters he sees three red dots with right eye and two green with the other eye and 4 (2 red, 1 green, 1 white) with both eyes. If the squinting patient sees four dots only it means he is having harmonious abnormal retinal correspondence but it is unusual for this anomalous binocular response to be appreciated at the normal distance of the test. If diplopia occurs so that five lights are appreciated, then the prisms are put in front of one eye base out or base in according to the type of deviation to eliminate diplopia. If the strength of the prism required to eliminate diplopia is equal to the angle of squint measured objectively then there is normal retinal correspondence. If it is less, there is unharmonious abnormal retinal correspondence.

Projected after Image Test

Both pupils of the patient were fully dilated and then a graticule having slit was put vertically in the project scope and then it was projected on the eye for twenty seconds. Now the graticule was rotated by 90°, i.e. kept horizontally and it was projected on the fovea of the leading eye for next twenty seconds. Then the patient was asked to look at the intermittently illuminated white screen to facilitate the after images and asked to draw the after images. If patient drew complete cross, he was declared to have normal retinal correspondence. If on the other hand he drew after image symmetrical cross or incomplete cross the patient was declared as having abnormal retinal correspondence. There patients who appreciated only vertical or horizontal after image, had suppression of one eye.

Bifoveal Correspondence Test

This is one of the most dissociating tests to determine retinal correspondence. In this test one eye was dilated with drosyn and the patient was asked to fix a small spotlight situated at 6 meters distance with the other eye.

Then by the projectoscope, using the after graticule, this star was projected on the fovea of the dilated eye and the patient was asked if he can see the star superimposed over the spotlight. If so, then normal retinal correspondence was declared in that case. If the patient unable to see the star over the spotlight but away from the spotlight then abnormal retinal correspondence was declared. If patient was unable to see the star and spotlight simultaneously, it indicated suppression of one eye.

Maddox Wing Test

Maddox wing test is also a useful test for binocular projection at a near distance while liking through the two holes, left eye sees the figures while the right eye sees arrow. If in the presence of squint the allow points at zero it shows that harmonious type of abnormal retinal correspondence is present. If the measurement of the angle by Maddox wing is less than in measured objectively, it means there is unharmonious abnormal retinal correspondence.

Maddox Rod Test

While we are determining the retinal correspondence the Maddox rod test records the subjective response of the patient, while the objective angle is determined by the prism and convertest, when objective response is zero in presence of manifest squint, shows there is harmonious abnormal retinal correspondence. If subjective response is less than the objective angle means unharmonious type. If it is equal to the objective one there is normal correspondence.

Diplopia Test

In diplopia test, the patient is asked to fix a small light source. Before this objective angle of squint is determined by the prism cover test or by synoptophore. Then a red glass is placed in front of one eye and green in front of the other eye. He will as a rule readily see two light, one red another white. In normal correspondence the direction and amount of separation of two light corresponds to the amount of deviation. If there is unharmonious abnormal retinal correspondence then the separation of the two image will be smaller than angle of squint. There would be no separation in harmonious type of abnormal retinal correspondence. Diplopia test is easily performed, even in small children, but patient often shows suppression on this test and this difficulty can be overcome to come extent by:

a. Putting red filter in front of eye which patient habitually used for fixation
b. A prism may be placed base up or base down (5 to 10 prism diopter) in front of one eye. This displaces the image above or below the region of elective suppression.

MANAGEMENT

Through ARC represents an abnormal reflex development which is capable of considerable degree of fixity and is an obstacle to the development or NRC and true fusion but it does provide a from of binocular cooperation that leads to a reasonable range of fusional amplitude (through anomalous) often and a harmonious ARC is often a highly satisfactory substitute for the normal sensory relationship of the two eyes through perverted and inferior to bifoveal fixation among to the poor resolution provided at the eccentric retinal point and thus through ARC cannot contribute significantly to the binocular image to give rise to "fine stereopsis" but when the deviation is small as in "microtropia" it does give rise to a "coarse stereopsis" never the less if the eyes are in favorable position from the cosmetic point of view, a harmonious ARC provides a useful degree of binocularity which makes the development of dense amblyopia less likely and tends to stabilize the position of eyes throughout life so that a consecutive divergence in esotropia becomes a rarity. If ARC is found to be present it is desirable to discover the extent to which it has developed fixity. It may be unstable and variable and thus amenable to treatment or it may be stable, constant and difficulty to eradicate. It is necessary to test the patient's power of fusion and if fusion pictures can be joined without difficulty the range of fusion can be tested on provided both control are visible presence of a range of fusion in a patient with ARC indicates a well-grounded perverted reflex which has been conditioned by time and usage in much the same way as a normal reflex. Presence of week stereoscopic vision demonstrable with large slides which requires peripheral fusion usually indicates a harmonious type of ARC. A well-established harmonious ARC carries a poor prognostic significance for treatment when treating patients with ARC it is essential to realize that not only one is aiming to overcome an abnormal reflex but one that has become accepted as correct with regard to the body although ocularly incorrect, so aim must be at establishing normal projection (binocular and uniocular) not only in relation to eyes but also to the body. Before reestablishing NRC it is essential to eradicate the ARC present which can be persued with two fold aims of treatment, *viz* (i) the further development and consolidation of ARC is prevented by obstructing abnormal binocular stimulus, which can be achieved by use of occlusion, orthoptic and surgical treatment as also by prism therapy, (ii) to attempt overcoming the present ARC and to restore normal correspondence and projection, (iii) when the decision is to consolidate the condition of ARC , attempts are made to make ARC usally alternative to normal binocular function by suitable orthoptic exercises the aim of treatment should be to improve the anomalous fusion range, to increase peripheral(anomalous) stereoscopic sense and to develop power of binocular convergence.

Treatment Modalities Available and their Scope

Occlusion Therapy

An ARC is a binocular condition so occlusion of one or other eye as a passive from of therapy serves the dual purpose of presentation of ARC by arresting its onward progress by interrupting the continued stimulating of noncorresponding points and curatively it also serves to reduce the stability of ARC, and to get better results it requires very often to be combinded with other form of treatment of ARC and continued uninterruptly and discarded only if it fails to serve its purpose after being given reasonably long period of trial. The place of occlusion in preoperative period is accepted by many surgeons to be helpful in breaking the ARC, but postoperative occlusion is advocated when the residual squint is seen to gradually increase in time in an attempt to reestablish the previous angle of anomaly.

Orthoptic Treatment

Stage I

a. Full correction of refractive error under complete cycloplegia
b. As already discussed, conventional occlusion to avoid stimulation of noncorresponding points and to stimulate anatomical fovea.

Stage II: Stimulation of the fovea once the vision in the amblyopic eye was sufficient to appreciate the foveal slide on the synoptophore, the patient was given stimulation of normal fovea by stimulating at the objective angle.

Method of stimulating at the objective angle: The objective angle was measured by the simultaneous foveal perception slides and the tubes were set at the objective angle. The automatic flashing device was switched on in front of the amblyopia eye stimulation was given from 10 to 15 minutes. (A careful observation is necessary to avoid any chance of using the abnormal retinal points. This can be done by drawing the patient's concentration to the fixation object by taping the picture in the fixing eye now and then and checking the objective angle).

a. Bi-kinetic retinal stimulation was performed using simultaneous foveal perception slides, deeping the tubes at the objective angle and the patient looking straight ahead, he was asked to superimpose the picture.
b. Appreciation of an after-image of symmetrical cross. This was done twice a day for 15-20 minutes for each sitting even while the conventional occlusion was being continued. As a result of the above stimulation, the angle of anomaly was reduced neared to normal.
c. In cases of gross amblyopia, appreciation of Hadinger's brushes was helpful both in improving the visual acuity and strengthening the normal fovea.

   A cross after image was produced fixing eye and the Hadinger's brush placed in front of the amblyopic eye. Patient was advised to superimpose the brush in the center of the cross after image. Failure to appreciate the brush is due to any organic lesion of the macular area.

Stage III: It is the stage where the objective and subjective angles are equal. At this stage antisuppression and fusional exercise were given using simultaneous foveal perception slides or Mayou slides in the synoptophore. Chasing, and in and out exercises were carried out. Fusional reserve and fusional range were exercised by fusional slides of foveal size with vertical controls.

Home Exercises

Cherioscopic tracing was advised as a home antisuppression exercises and also Kodak Wratten Gelating Filter Red No. 92 (wavelength of which is 600 u) was used in front of the amblyopic eye along with the continued conventional occlusion which allowed only the stimulation of the macular area. This gave the best result in improving the visual acuity and strengthening the anatomical fovea.

Prismotherapy

Principles and aims of prism therapy in ARC. They are: (i) to secure a state of sensory orthropsia of the eye so that simultaneous stimulation of the fovea and other corresponding points of the two retinal is attended in natural condition of seeing in everyday life, but treatment period may extend between 2-8 months of even 18 months, requires frequent careful observation during this period with frequent change of power of prism correction, (ii) to foster the development and consolidation of bifoveal relationship, it very often requires to be combined with other requires to be combined with other measure like orthoptics and surgery when indicated to obtain a final motor balance between the eyes to ensure that fusion is maintained through the creation of sensory orthotropsia by prismotherapy is unlikely to be followed by a spontaneous elimination of the deviation except perhaps in small angle esotropia, (iii) As a rule, the prismatic correction is applied equally by dividing the power between the two eyes the base of will obviously on the type of the strength of prismatic correction depends on the judgment whether to correct exactly or over correct the deviation.

Indications and contraindications of prismotherapy: Elimination of amblyopia if present is an essential prerequisite for effective prismotherapy. Prismotherapy is also useless in (i) congenital squint, alternating of uniocular, when the innate capacity for fusion is even potentially absent, (ii) in the presence of intractable amblyopia, (iii) when for any reason a satisfactory state of motor balance cannot be obtained by any means.

It is suitable in young children with sensory mechanism relatively plastic or in when the ARC has not been firmly entrenched and it is often useful also in tacking a persistent postoperative paradoxical diplopia in an adult if functional cause for it can be ruled out preoperative prismotherapy may appear more reasonable to establish bifoveal vision except when the squints more than 35 to 40D or in the presence of marked degree of incomitances in the horizontal or vertical plane so that angle of deviation is variable. Postoperative prismotherapy is helpful to secure and promote bifoveal stimulation during the transitory period after surgery or the relieve persistent post-operative diplopia in adults.

Surgical Treatment of ARC

It should be emphasized that the best treatment of anomalous retinal correspondence is surgery. Identifying the presence of ARC inform the surgeon that the patient will experience diplopia immediately after surgery presuming the eye alignment has been changed sufficiently to move the image of the object of regard outside the suppression scotoma. Postoperative paradoxical diplopia is more readily accepted in children than in adults.

In cases where the angle is large, the preliminary surgical correction of the angle helps easy carrying out of the orthoptic treatment usually surgery was performed into cases when the presence of ocular deviation was obvious and there were complains of diplopia and abnormal head posture. Results may follow surgical treatment of a case of esotropia with ARC (i) NRC with binocular single vision in which case, the retinal correspondence should be consolidated by further orthoptic treatment (ii) there may be a small residual deviation but with development of NAC. Further orthoptic treatment and/or further surgical treatment should be undertaken within a short interval of time in order to eradicate the deviation, (iii) the ocular appearance may be improved but ARC may be still present. Although no further orthoptic treatment is necessary. Such cases need not be kept under observation. If there is indication that NRC can be developed, further orthoptic treatment should be considered immediately, (iv) tertiary correspondence may occur in which case no further treatment is indicated, (v) the deviation may revert to the original angle of squint. Orthotic treatment including occlusion is indicated for a limited period and it may be necessary.

Postoperatively a course of orthoptic exercises were carried out in improving the binocular functions and fusional reserve.

16 Amblyopia

The term *amblyopia* is derived from 2 Greek words Aubus meaning blunt and Wu meaning vision, i.e. blunt vision.

Amblyopia is a condition of diminished visual acuity which is not associated with any structural abnormality or disease of media, fundi or visual pathway and which is not overcome by the correction of the refractive error. It is generally accepted that uniocular amblyopia is present if the best corrected vision in one eye is at least 2 lines poorer on the Snellen chart than the other eye and no organic pathology is seen.

CLASSIFICATION

Chavasse (1939) classified amblyopia mainly into two groups.

Amblyopia of arrest: This occurs due to the deviation of the eye during plastic period of macular development, i.e. from birth to six years, so that the macular development in the deviated eye is arrested.

Amblyopia of extinction: This occurs when the visual acuity is already present but is lost through inhibition and disuse. This portion of amblyopia can be recovered, if the treatment is instituted the right time.

It is felt that since information above the retinal correspondence is of more value than any other thing in a case of amblyopia. So, amblyopia is classified according to the type of retinal correspondence. Accordingly cases of amblyopia has been classified as follows:

I. Amblyopia with strabismus and normal retinal correspondence.
II. High grade amblyopia with strabismus and abnormal retinal correspondence.
III. Moderate amblyopia with strabismus and abnormal retinal correspondence.
IV. Amblyopia with strabismus and mixed retinal correspondence. Mixed retinal correspondence means functional association in which

correspondence is not firmly established so that it may vary with the method or time of testing.

V. Amblyopia with strabismus due to anisometropia, with, normal retinal correspondence.

VI. Amblyopia without demonstrable strabismus due to spontaneous reduction of a manifest deviation.

VII. Amblyopia which is usually due to congenital cataract and is said to be classical type of amblyopia exanopsia. Amblyopia is customarily divided into following groups or categories:

Congenital Amblyopia

It may involve one or both eyes. It can be of the following three types:

a. Organic amblyopia
   Receptor amblyopia or due to central hemorrhage
b. Amblyopia secondary to nystagmus
   i. Latent nystagmus
   ii. Manifest micronystagmus
c. Amblyopia secondary to congenital achromotopia.

Ametropic Amblyopia

It occur in one or both eyes in children and adults who have significant refractive errors and have not worn their glasses previously. The vision remained poor and the retina continued to function at a subnormal levels for years. There cases are mostly of high hypermetropia or astigmatism. When prescribed spectacles in adult age, they rarely show an immediate improvement of vision. However, a regular use of correct spectacles for months or years may bring about a marked visual improvement without any other therapy.

Anisometropia Amblyopia

In there cases one eye has got a normal or near normal visual acuity and the other has a high refractive error most commonly hypermetropia, some times a high astigmatism and occasionally in high myopia where the far paint is so close to the eyes that it is not practical to use the eye even for close work. These cases specially that of the hypermetropic or astigmatic group mostly maintain straight eye and therefore a central or foveal fixation and at least some binocular function. In anisometropia the visual objects imaged on the two foveas are identical but of different sharpness, or if the anisometropia is corrected of different size (aniseikonia). Inhibition thus occurs to keep a blurred image from the more ametropic eye from interfering with perception of sharp image from the fellow eye. The retinal images of different nature percent an obstacle to fusion therefore, anisometropia may be quite often associated with secondary strabismus.

Strabismus Amblyopia

In this condition there is a reduced visual acuity in one eye in patients with strabismus or a history of strabismus without ophthalmoscopically demonstrable anomalies of the fundus.

It is an active suppression of the reception of stimuli from certain parts of the retina by the brain. This means that the higher visual centers and related areas responsible for the reception of stimuli and perception of an image start disregarding the stimulesent by one or more areas of retina usually there are such two areas in the squinting eye, i.e. the macula which is responsible for confusion and another more peripheral area which is responsible for diplopia. This process of active inhibition of stimuli in brain is facultative in early stage but becomes obligatory in late stage. Continued suppression of the stimuli from the macular area leads to amblyopia. Which it seems reasonable to is a result of pure active inhibition in early stages but there in a combination of both active and passive processes in late or well-established cases of amblyopia, i.e. a factor of disuse becomes superimposed upon the continued and constant active inhibition, in a matter of months or more usually years (5). Stimulus Deprivation Amblyopia (Amblyopia Exanopsia) — If occurs in children with congenital total cataract, complete ptosis of corneal opacitis, etc. The amblyopia is because of lack of stimulation during the formative period. The exact nature of the lesion is not clear, head tilting is known about the site and mechanism of this defect but this amblyopia differs at least clinically from amblyopia in strabismus and anisometropia by its irreversibility and occasional bilateral occurrence. Generally visual outcome is less favorable in children with complete congenital cataract than in those with partial congenital cataract, even when the ocular media are perfectly transparent postoperatively. In some of there cases foveal hypoplasia has been assure to be the cause for the visual loss,especially if poor vision is associated with microophthalmos or other congenital anomalies. In other the history clearly indicates that disuse may have indeed been a fact in producing amblyopia.

Meridional Amblyopia

Visual acuity in astigmatism may vary according to the degree of astigmatism while astigmatism of lower degree does not affect visual acuity, higher degree may be associated with reduced vision, which may be correctable with correction of the refractive error. If, however, if may remain uncorrected for a long time, it may be associated with amblyopia. Any of there subjects may have better vision in one meridian than in the other corresponding to the axis of astigmatism even after wearing full optical correction. This condition is called Meridional amblyopia. The condition has been known clinically for a long time. In meridional amblyopia, contrast sensitivity function is reduced, neural element that process spatial frequencies are affected by meridional amblyopia. Retinal sensitivity has also been found to be reduced in the amblyopia meridian in cases of meridional amblyopia. Meridional amblyopia also found in subjects who developed astigmatism secondary to soft tissue anomalies of the orbit in their early life.

HERIDITY IN AMBLYOPIA

Amblyopia which so often accompanies concomitant squint and refractive errors is not genetically determined but because it is only a secondary characteristic inheritance may be associated only because of inheritance of myopia, hypermetropia or concomitant squint.

Ocular Dominance

Dominance may be defined as physiological pre-eminence, priority or preferential activity of one of any anatomically similar bilateral pair of structure in the body for example the hands, the feet, the eyes, ears and two cerebral hemisphere, ocular dominance is the term used for the physiological superiority of one type of an individual over the other eye during binocular through both eyes are anatomically and optically identical. The dominant eye possesses a greater sense of clarity, sharpness of outline and detail and refinement of discrimination. The role of ocular dominance in amblyopia, squint has gained importance. In treatment of amblyopia, cases with crossed dominance showed greater benefit from occlusion because the amblyopic eye is encouraged to be used better. The functional status of the fellow dominant in amblyopia also needs attention. It has been pointed out that the fellow dominant eve is also not a normal eye as compared to control normal eye with binocular fixation.

The changes related to ocular dominance can be demonstrated more clearly in layer IV of the striate cortex.

VISUAL ACUITY IN AMBLYOPIA

From a practical clinical stand point, a difference in vision of two lines on visual acuity chart is frequently used as a diagnostic criteria for amblyopia. Neutral density filters produce a profound reduction in vision in eyes with central retinal lesions and glaucoma whereas "the vision of the eyes with functional amblyopia is not reduced by such filters and occasionally even slightly improves.

Many patients with amblyopia are capable of discriminating rather small visual acuity symbols when they are presented singly against a uniform ground, whereas when there symbols are presented in a row, as on a visual acuity chart, they must be larger for a patient to be able to recognize them with amblyopia eye. Thus, most amblyopia eyes seen to have two. Acuities, which could be designated as line acuity, or 'Snellen' acuity and single E acuity. This is known as crowding phenomenon. At the completion of treatment, presence or absence of crowding phenomenon has significant prognostic value.

ACCOMMODATION IN AMBLYOPIA

Visual acuity in near fixation is better than in distance fixation in a number of amblyopics. There is improvement in the fixation pattern of the amblyopia eye in downward gaze and there is a weakness of accommodation of the amblyopia eye compared with that of the normally sighted fellow eye. The third of amblyopic patients have reduced accommodation in their defective eye. Accommodation in a case of amblyopia was very low both for near and distance as compared with control cases. However, it improved significantly immediately often completion of treatment by penalization. Retinal threshold and sensitivity—There is a decreased sensitivity of the foveal cones in amblyopia. Flicker fusion threshold of the foveal area of patients of amblyopia is considerably depressed. A functional defect of the foveal cones would be responsible for a reduced visual acuity.

Phenomenon of Contest

The ability of strabismus amblyopia eye to differentiate contours in varying degree of luminance of the background and found that higher degree of contrast than normal is required at ordinary levels of illumination but in a dim light no significant difference between the ability of the two eyes are demonstrable. In organic amblyopia retina behaves normally in this respect.

Pupillometer Anomaly

Macular area has the highest pupillometer sensitivity in normal eyes, whereas in amblyopia eyes the pupillometer sensitivity was greater peripherally than centrally studies have also shown that pupil of the amblyopic eye on an average is 0.5 mm larger than the normal eye.

Dark Adaptation

There is slight delay in the dark adaptation of the amblyopic eye due to raised, threshold of the rods. But it has been shown by various workers that the visual acuity of an amblyopic eye may increase almost to the level usually achieved by the normal eye, in dim illumination and sometimes there may even be a slight improvement in the vision of the amblyopic eye when the illumination is reduced. This shows that the defect lies in the photopic vision restricted to the cones in the central area while the peripheral retina remains normal.

Color Sense

Usually, it is normal but minor defects may occur in severe cases.

Light Sense

There is no difference is the light sense of the amblyopia and of the normal fellow eye. The amblyopic eye yields the typical responses and typical differences between center and periphery expected from normal eye. The entire apparatus of simple light perception is virtually normal in the amblyopic eye.

Fixation Movement—Patterns

In dark adopted states, the amblyopic eye exhibits remarkably steady central fixation, even if the eye in ordinary conditions showed eccentric or wordering fixation.

Normally, a saccadic movement occurs when an eye changes fixation point. In conditions of light this saccadic movement is irregular with fine oscillations in an amblyopic eye while in dark adaptation the amblyopic eye moves normally.

Central fixation in constantly squinting eye may be lost in infant within 6 and 8 weeks 5 and 6 months, at 18 months of age and so on, but after the age of 6 it is never lost eccentric fixation (nonfoveolar) and no fixation nonfoveolar fixation may be parafoveolar (between the foveola and the macula), paramacular (outside but close to the edge of the macular) or peripheral some where between the edge of the macula and the disk and occasionally even beyond the disk, eccentric fixation develops on the basic of an anomalous retinal correspondence and the eccentric fixation area becomes associated with the principle visual direction Mechanism of development of eccentric fixation is a form of sensory and motor adaptation of visual processes in strabismus.

Amblyopic Scotoma

To avoid confusion and diplopia during simultaneous activity of the two eyes, two types of suppression occur:

i. Suppression of the area of the retina of the squinting eye which has same projection as the fixing fovea.
ii. Suppression of the area of the retina of the squinting eye corresponding to the angle of squint to allow free play to the fixing fovea at the fixation point.

ERG1: Studies showed no consistent difference in the wave forms between normal and amblyopic eyes.

VER: Shows slight reduction of amplitude in amblyopia and that too not consistent with the degree of amblyopia. Latency has been shown to be increased in the amblyopic eyes.

All these visual responses of the amblyopic eye do not imply that the amblyopic mechanism is retina itself. The abnormality arises from the fact that the fovea of the amblyopia eyes in themselves give normal scotopic responses at photopic luminance level.

SCREENING OF AMBLYOPIC-STERCO-ACUITY

I. *Stero test*: Sometimes it may not be possible to differentiate between amblyopia and heterotropia due to some false visual clues in this test.
II. *Random dot E test*: To overcome false result in Titmus test. This test is simple to perform and gives a pass or fail response. It can also be quantituted by increasing the testing distance from the patient.

III. *TNO test*: Provide quick assessment and some further clues in amblyopia.

Out of all there tests, Random test is more reliable than other methods.

IV. *Dynamic stereopsis test*: This device is easier to use and interpret correctly than random dot stereogram.

On the basis of value of contrast images on stereopsis and normal binocular vision there is a relationship between stereopsis and binocular cortical neurons. Recovery of binocularity has been minimum.

PATHOGENESIS OF AMBLYOPIA

There is a considerable diversity of opinions regarding the seat of inhibition in a case of amblyopia.

1. The retina: In some amblyopia eyes there is a malorientation of retinal receptors. Frequent retinal hemorrhages of neonates defects of retinal ganglion cells, sustained or cells in the area central is of the retina, provide the physiological basis of high visual acuity. Amblyopia is a functional loss of 'X' cells due to inappropriate stimulations of the fovea by habitually blurred images during the critical period of development. It has been supported by experiments on kittens with surgically produced squint or penalization. In unilateral amblyopia as in uniocular squint or anisometropia, the X-cells would be inadequately stimulated as both produce blurred images. Amblyopia retinal ganglion cells cause a slight in ocular dominance in the cortex.

No changes in the size of the parafoveal or peripheral retinal ganglion cells were found in the eye, which was sutured. Only one case, where suture was left-from one to two year of age showed decrease in the density of the parafoveal ganglion cells but the peripheral portion were normal. Form there experimental studies we can reclassify amblyopia in two basic types, abnormal binocular interaction amblyopia and stimulus deprivation with abnormal binocular interaction amblyopia from vision deprivation is the exclusive cause of unilateral amblyopia as caused by unilateral congenited cataract, corneal opacities, bilateral high hypermetropia. Unilateral amblyopia in cases of strabismus, anisometropia and unilateral cataract is caused by a combination of visual deprivation and abnormal binocular interaction.

2. According to another view the seat of inhibition in amblyopia is in central nervous system. Relative lowering of the pupillary responses to light in amblyopia eyes suggested that inhibition originated in the cortex

and was projected so as to suppress the activity of retina. In amblyopia vision the entire apparatus of light perception and spatial localization is normal, while form vision suffers, particularly in bright light. The complete removal of occipital lobes results in virtually complete loss of pattern and object vision with little loss in the capacity to react to light to discriminate brightness.

Thus, pattern vision is cortical and the other visual function are subcortical. Amblyopia, therefore appears to be the cortical inhibition of the highest function of pattern vision without improvement of the lower functions of the light sense and spatial projection. There is decreased sensitivity of the foveal cones. Flicker-Fusion threshold of the foveal area of patients with amblyopia is considerably depressed. When fluctuation of retinal illuminance with change of pupil diameter are prevented with an artificial pupillary aperature the critical flickes frequency for the center of the field is lower in amblyopia eye than in the normal eye. It is observed that reduction of foveal cones sensitivity was much less than the reduction of visual acuity in such eyes. Therefore, it appears in probable that functional defect of the foveal cones would be responsible for a reduced visual acuity. In case of amblyopia, there is a possible existence of visual agnosis. Amblyopia eye is not at its best under photopic condition but it shows a relative improvement of its function its function under mesopic condition. Light adopted amblyopic eyes were characterized by unsteadiness and jerky movement during fixation. The unsteadiness and jerky movements were seen to disappear entirely when the amblyopic eyes were dark adopted. Amblyopic eye showed relatively improved or normal function under reduced illumination in contrast to pathologically amblyopic eye suggesting that mechanism which operates in strabismus amblyopia must differ from that in the presence of organic lesion.

The spatial summation (functions) of the amblyopic eyes at the fovea was considerably higher in the light adopted state than in the normal fellow eyes. There is a high contrast requirement of the amblyopic eye at high luminances clearly differing from normal eye. A study experimental amblyopia in retinas of cat showed atrophy in the corpus geniculation and functional disturbances in the cortex. By cutting one medial rectus in kitten, alternating strabismus developed. These kitten developed functional disturbances. The number of cortical cells driven by both eyes decreased from 80 to 20%. This would seen to indicate that the seat of suppression is to be found in the cerebral cortex.

The functions integuity of the visual system may depend not only on the adequacy of afferent impulse activity but also an interrelationship and possible interaction of the input received by one eye.

Optometer responses and adjustments resulting from visual stimule apparently take place after relay of visual impulses, from area 17 (striate area) to area 18 + 19 (parastriate area). If there is rivalry between the two eyes requiring suppression the conflict must be resolved at this level, and as a result in some instances an altered fixation or optometer response pattern will also emerge in the final resolution of the conflict. It has been shown experimentally in monkeys that no inhibitory pattern leader into area 17 proper, therefore the incoming visual impulse much reach area 18 and 19 before any adjustment, either motor or sensory, can take place. All other cortical association pathways having to do with vision and visual responses channel into this area as well.

In EEG, with alternate stimulation of the normal and amblyopic eyes there is a characteristic difference. The normal response is blocking of the alpha rhythm and this occurred when the normal eye was stimulated. When the amblyopic eye was stimulated, no suppression or alpha activity occurred when the vision was below 20/70. They concluded that these, difference in cerebral response would place the seat of the defect in hemispheres rather than in the retina. There is abnormal alpha rhythm in amblyopia.

The recent finding from a study of experimental amblyopic in the rhesus monkey, where amblyopia of varying degree was produced by unilateral lid closure of artificial esotropia, suggested that only a small number of neurons were driven from the deprived or the deviated eye with less severe amblyopia many neurons received input from that eye. Invisual cortex normally 80% of the cells in the visual cortex are binocular, i.e. they respond to stimule from either eye and 20% cells are monocular. Number of binocular driven cells in visual cortex were significantly decreased as also the monocular driven cells that could be activated through the deprived eye.

3. The optic nerve-amblyopia may be caused by occurrence of hemorrhages in the optic nerve in the newborn or by delay in normal process of mylenization of the nerve fibers.

4. Lateral geniculate body is other possible site suggested of visual pathway for the site and cause of amblyopia. Amblyopia, which does not improve might be due to atrophy of disuse in the cells of lateral

geniculate nucleus which depend on both retinal and cortical activity for then continued vitality. There is a significant reduction of cell section areas in all layers of lateral geniculate nucleus that received input from the deprived or esotropic eye cell, shrinkage is observed in the lateral geniculate nucleus with the number of cortical neurons that responded to stimulation from the deprived or esotropic eye. In strabismus the cells sizes were decreased only in the binocularly in everted portion of LGK and no effect was seen on monocular interaction of the sole amblyogenic factor in cases of squint.

INCIDENCE OF AMBLYOPIA

The incidence of amblyopia is high enough in general population to pose an important economic problem. In uniocular visual loss 66% cases are due to amblyopia. The incidence of strabismus with amblyopia is 2.2%.

TREATMENT OF FUNCTIONAL AMBLYOPIA

Various methods of treatment have been advocated in amblyopia.

1. Correction of refractive error
2. Occlusion
3. Red filter treatment
4. Penalization
5. Prisms
6. Pleoptics
7. Pharmacologic therapy
8. Minimal occlusion
9. CAM vision—stimulator treatment
10. Rapid Autoflashing
11. Levodopa with minimal occlusion
12. Orthoptic treatment.

Correction of Refractive Error

One of the most important steps in the management of any case of amblyopia is retinoscopy under full cycloplegia and prescription of suitable glasses wherever indicated. However, there are certain specific indication are:

1. Accommodation squint in strabismus amblyopia
2. Anisometropic amblyopia
3. Ametropic amblyopia.

In children below the age of 5 years, full objective correction as determined by retinoscopy should be prescribed. Above that age where full cooperation of the patient is available, the power of the glasses prescribed should be such that it gives the maximum correction of squint and the best visual acuity for distance near.

Occlusion

The concept behind patching of good eye (Conventional occlusion) is to force the amblyopic eye to develop normal visual acuity by constant use. Conventional is not advocated in cases of eccentric fixation because it may intensify and establish eccentric fixation. In such cases, inverse occlusion is advised conventional occlusion of the fixating eye during all working hours, regardless of the fixation behavior of the amblyopic eye. However, care should be taken to avoid occlusion amblyopia when occluding at ages between birth and the age five years. Occlusion of the sound eye has been carried out a 3 to 1 or 1 to 1 basis in first year or second year of age to prevent occlusion amblyopia (i.e. amblyopia eye is occluded every fourth or fifth day) occlusion is continued until visual acuity is equal in both eyes. If there is no improvement after a three or four month period of constant treatment it is discontinued. Instead of patch soft contact lens (occluder) can be used.

Advantages of Occlusion of Amblyopia Eye

1. Occlusion of the amblyopic eye accustoms the child to wearing occlusion before there is frightening loss of vision.
2. The spatial localization of the retina of the squinting eye become more normal under the occlusion, so that occlusion is changed to the fixing eye, the chance of false projection or uniocular deplopia are greatly reduced.
3. Visits to clinic need not be frequent. These difficulties of transport, finance and use of the orthoptic test's time are overcome.

Disadvantages

1. The treatment is very lengthy. Parents and child find the wearing of occlusion for long tedious and unless there is a noticeable improvement the patients are noncooperative.
2. The final visual improvement is frequently not dramatic, particularly if prolonged occlusion on the fixing eye has been carried out previously.

3. For the best results it is still necessary to start occlusion, under 5 years of age.

Therefore, the present trend to prescribe occlusion of the sound eye in cases of children below the age of six years whether eccentric fixation exists or not. Above that age, squinting eye should be occluded in the presence of eccentric fixation. This would cut down the total time of occlusion and duration of treatment, if successful.

Practical Application of Recent Concept

i. Occlusion therapy acts by removing the inhibitory stimulate to the amblyopic eye that arise from stimulation of fixing eye concept of occlusion amblyopia should not mean that occlusion therapy is dangerous up to 6 years of age. One the contrary, it is more effective when started at the younger age.
ii. Occlusion should as a rule, always be complete and constant during all working hours. Partial occlusion may cause abnormal binocular interaction.
iii. Prolonged occlusion at early age may cause occlusion amblyopia, so eye may be patched on 3 to 1 day rhythm during first year of life, 4 to 1 day during second year and late on it is prolonged with frequent checkups. During the period when patch is removed from fixing eye, amblyopic eye should be patched, so that abnormal binocular interaction do not become active.
iv. In correction of gross anisometropia contact lenses should be given, to reduce the risk of aniseikonic amblyopia.

Red Filter Treatment

For treatment of amblyopia with eccentric fixation, Brinker and Kotz (1963) suggested occlusion of the sound eye and application of red filter that excludes wavelength shorter than 640 mm, on the spectacle frame before the amblyopic eye.

Principle

The retina contains the light sensitive cells, the rods and cones. The fovea consists only of cones and concentration of cones decreases towards the periphery while the concentration of rod increases. If a patient has got foveal fixation he has cone fixation. But if the fixation is eccentric beyond the immediate parafoveal region, he may be assured to have rod fixation. If light is prevented from stimulating rod but it is allowed to stimulate cones, then presentably the patient will fix with the area of the retina having greatest concentration of cones, i.e. fovea.

A filter is used which is of such optical qualities that is transmits only light, which stimulates the cones, and no light to which the rods might be sensitive, such a filter is the Kodak No. 92 Red-Wratten-filter.

Advantages

i. This filter method requires less time of both the orthoptist and the patient, attendances being weekly instead of daily.
ii. Cooperation is required from the patient apart from wearing the filter occlusion. This enables treatment to be carried out on very young children.
iii. No extensive equipment is necessary.

Disadvantages

i. This red filter is not suitable to be worn for long time as it quickly becomes scratched and cracked; a substitute filter has however bear found in the Huby-Kodalaid filter which closely resembles the Kodak in optical qualities but is made of strong material.
ii. Many patients will not tolerate the total occlusion of good eye, it is therefore suggested that the red filter may be worn for increasing period each day and that the eccentrically fixing eye should be totally occluded at other time.

   Treatment should be continued for nine months to one year before a case is considered incapable of being improved with red filter.

Penalization

Penalization (means punishment or inhibition) defines as cycloplegia with atropine and over correction of the fixating eye with spectacles. The principle of the penalization is to blue the near vision of the fixating eye by atropine so that the patient uses amblyopic eye for near work.

There are following methods of penalization:

A. Penalization for near
B. Penalization for distance
C. Total penalization
D. Selective penalization
E. Alternating distance penalization.

Advantages

i. Penalization is essentially a kind of mild or partial occlusion of the good eye which have cosmetic benefit and avoids occlusion amblyopia.
ii. It is applicable in early cases of amblyopia and in cases of amblyopia where visual acuity is better than 20/200.
iii. It is helpful in cases of amblyopia with latent component of congenital hystagmus.

However, the inhibitory influence of the sound eye is not eliminated in penalization.

Minimal Occlusion

Here the child wears a totally opaque patch for only 20-30 minutes a day, during which he plays some kind of visually demanding game which demands much concentration. The task is as fine and difficult as he is able to undertake.

CAM Vision—Stimulator Treatment

Principles—This is a physiologically bases new method of treatment for amblyopia. The new technique consisted of occlusion of the functional eye for only 7 to 10 minutes, during which the amblyopia, eye views a very powerful stimulus of slowly rotating high contrast square wave gatings of the highest spatial frequencies appreciated by the patient.

CAM vision stimulator is neutrophysiologically based. All cells in the visual cortex of the cat and monkey are specifically sensitive to the orientation of a bar, edge or grating stimulus. This discovery caused a revolution in the field of amblyopia research and attempts were made to show that human visual system was similarly organized. There are at least two different types of ganglion cells in the cat retina. They showed that 'X' type neuron behaves linearly. The finding that some of the hardwars of the visual system was behaving sufficiently linearly, led to further new work in psychophysics and neurophysiology. Long exposive to a grating of given spatial frequency (Number of cycle per degree of visual angle) and orientation reduces the sensitivity of the visual system at that spatial frequency and orientation. By this indirect method they were able to define spatial frequency sensitivity of individual channels or discrete set of channels. We can treat visual neurons tuned filters for spatial frequencies in same way as auditory physiologist treat auditory neurons as turned filters for sound frequencies. Some amblyopia have decreased visual acuity for optotypes, but can exhibit normal contrast sensitivity function. This means that neurons for detecting each spatial frequency present and able to signal the presence of a grating target with normal sensitivity. On the basis of these observation a stimulus should be employed to activate each set of neurones in turn, and the obvious way of doing this is to rotate a high contract black and white striped pattern (grating) slowly through 360°. This would then activate all orientationally selective neuron in turn. Further, grating patterns of different spatial frequency would have to be rotated to activate each set of size dependent neurons.

CAM vision stimulates is an instrument developed one principles evolved by Professor Fergns Campbell, at Cambridge University. It consists of a box like device on which an appropriate grating due car, be placed over a lurn plate immediately behind a transparent plastic plate. The grating disk can be rotated at the rate of one revolution per minute, after connecting the instrument to electric supply. There are seven high contrast square wave gratings, circular in shape and of different spatial frequencies. Before starting the treatment the patient was shown the series of the gratings, after covering his normal eye. The widest stripe was presented first and he was asked to indicate the orientation of grating by pointing in the direction of the times. Thus the finest stripe he could see was determined. During the treatment, patient was shown the grating in sequences from the level spatial frequency to the highest special frequency he could see.

With normal eye occluded, patient was seated in front of the CAM vision stimulator. The first grating was placed on the turn table and than transparent plate was placed over it. The patient was engaged in pencil games (i.e. to draw pictures, circles or squares) on the plate, where the grating was relating. The patient was asked to hold his head as far away from the apparatus, as he could (preferably 28 cm). This procedure helped to concentrate fixation on the underlying stimulus, patient was also monitored constantly for his eye position and alertness to ensure? A high level of attention to the task one grating was rotated for 1-2 minutes and then next grading was placed over the turn lable. The total treatment session lasted for 10-14 minutes. Such patient received the grating stimulation individually. The patient was then sent home with his normal eye unoccluded.

Such treatment was administered on daily basis and visual acuity was assessed at weakly internals. The treatment was stopped if no improvement occurred at the end of 7 sessions. If vision improved, the treatment was continued till no further improvement occurred.

It may be the intense nature of visual tasks and concentrated eye hand coordination performed by the patient, which leads to the improvement of vision. Grading stimulation is slightly better than occlusion in improving visual acuity in anisometropic amblyopia with central fixation. CAM stimulation is a treatment of choice, it the long-term sound eye occlusion cannot be performed for any reason.

Autoflashing

By rapid flashing stimulation on synaptophore, stimulation of sound eye and minimal occlusion of the sound eye.

Usually, there is improvement in distant visual acuity in all patients ranging from one to three times on Snellen's chart. Clement Clark synaptophase (Model 2051) is usually used. It has got an automatic flashing device attached to its base one or both of the tubes can be intermittently illuminated. Patient was made to sit in front of synaptophore and his normal eye was occluded. Foveal/Paramacular perception slight was put in front of the amblyopia eye, depending upon its visual acuity lamp in tube in front of the patient was rapidly flashed after putting the dial setting on RAPID, and the patient was asked to concentrate on the target. The session lasted for 15 minutes and then the occluder before the normal eye was removed. Treatment was administered on daily basis visual acuity was assessed at the end of seven sessions. Treatment was stopped if there was no improvement. In cases, showing improvement, treatment was continued fill no further improvement in visual acuity occurred.

Prism

Use of prism is not much popular. Prisms have been used in combination with, occlusion therapy for the treatment of amblyopia with eccentric fixation. Usually ophthalmological use several prism that it base in for esotropia and base out for exotropia along with patient occlusion of sound eye with the help of neutral density fill.

Pleoptics (Gr. Pleos, full, Gr. Optikos, pertaining to sight)

Bangerter (1946) coined the term pleoptics which included all treatment of amblyopia by whatever method, including conventional, collision. Principle of Bangerter's method of treating amblyopia with eccentric fixation is to dazzle the eccentrically fixation retinal area with bright light while protecting the fovea, followed by intermittent stimulation of the macula with flashes of light, under direct observation of the therapist. Cuppers (1956, 1961) in his approach to treat eccentric fixation, attempted to reestablish, at least temporarily, the physiologic superiority of the fovea over retinal periphery with a modified ophthalmoscope (Euthyscope), fovea is protected with a black mask, retinal periphery including the area used for eccentric fixation is dazzled with bright light. A negative after-image is provoked and enhanced by flickering more illumination. The treatment is complimented by fixation exercised using. Haidinger brushes (coordinator) or a combination of Haindinger bruches and after images. However, this method is not possible. In its patients under 6 years of age as sustained concentration and cooperation is required.

This is a great controversies of over the efficiency of pleoptic treatment.

Pharmacologic Therapy

In some cases of strabismus amblyopia, there is improvement with small dose of strychnine. There is relatively good evidence that neuronal inhibit and within the visual cortex is mediated by inhibitory neurotransmitter, gamma-aminobutyric acid. The reveal of certain affects of visual deprivation can be observed by intravenous injection of Bicuculline and by enhancing neuronal plasticity by activating central norepinephrine system. Thus neurochemical reactivation of dormant visual connections or protection of the visual system against amblyopia may thus one day reverse or prevent amblyopia.

Levodopa/Carbidopa for Childhood Amblyopia

The neurotransmitter dopamine (DA) is involved in several visual functions. Visual deprivation decreases retinal DA concentration in chicken monkeys. In animals with deprivation amblyopia several studies suggest that neurotransmitters are involved in visual cortical plasticity and can release partial visual acuity in adult cats. By an action on D1 or D2 receptors. DA influences receptive field properties of retinal neurons, gap junction between horizontal cells, light adaptive movement between rods and cones and appears also to be involved in visual information processing to the brain. In human, light DA contents have been defected in amacrine and interplexi form cells. A physiological visual evoked potential and contact sensitivity in Parkinson's disease, which is characterized by a general dopamine deficiency, further more, levodopa administration increases the ERG- b-wave, selectively changes the amplitude of oscillatory potentials. An association between functional channels in the visual pathway (i.e. amblyopia) and neurotransmitter in the activity is strongly suggested by literature. From deprivation of chickens and occlusion of newborn infant monkey decreased retinal DA concentration. Other studies demonstrated that catecholamines and other neurotransmitters such as GABA, acetylcholine and glut a mats are involved in neuronal plasticity in deprivation amblyopia and can restore partial visual acuity in adult cats. It has been seen dopamine is present in the human retina paid also appears to involved in visual information processing; to brain, the dopaminergic effect cannot be localized to a specific part of the visual pathway. Levodopa, with a fixed dose combination of peripheral decarboxylase inhibitor (e.g. carbidopa) can temporarily improve visual acuity, contrast sensitivity and decrease scotoma size in amblyopia eye of children and adult.

The traditional treatment for amblyopia is ecclusion of the dominant eye and forced use of the amblyopia eye, when occlusion is first implemented on a child with active amblyopia, the success of occlusion therapy is dependent on compliance and, from a clinical perspective, compliance depends on the child's initial visual acuity in the amblyopic eye children with deep amblyopia, say worse than 20/100 are less likely to comply with occlusion than children with mild amblyopia when the child with deep amblyopia has his dominant eye occluded, he does not have any functional vision with the amblyopic eye, find it difficult to watch television, play grasses or do close work or home work. If levodopa/carbidopa can be used to improve visual acuity such the functional vision can be achieved by the amblyopic eye then compliance could be increased and success of occlusion therapy might be improved. It is believed that levodopa/carbidopa could be tolerated by children with amblyopia and support the possibility that levodopa/carbidopa could be used to augment occlusion therapy, older children and even adults could be benefitted with levodopa/carbidopa therapy 3 weeks of part time occlusion combined with levodopa/carbidopa can yield improved children and amblyopia adults, levodopa therapy is very encouraging and warrants further study.

Orthoptic Treatment

Immediately after completing one or the other form of the above treatment, the patient is given fusion exercises, The session lasts for 10 minutes as is administered on the daily basis fill the fusional amplitudes increases.

Home Exercises

During the period of treatment for amblyopia, patient is also asked to do some home exercises to stimulate vision in the amblyopic eye. These consisted of watching television, threading the needle and to read through a passage of newsprint of appropriate size at proper working distance. He is asked to spend about twenty-thirty minutes daily for these exercises.

17 *Aniseikonia*

In general, vision is a sensory function upon which depends the natural position of the objects that surrounds us. The spatial relationship of objects is known to us in two way through perceptive and stereoscopic sense. Perceptive sense is based on relative size, shape and positioning of the images of various subjects. Thus, if there is disparity in relative image size and shape, there will be defective spatial localization of the object.

The difference in relative size and shape of ocular image is termed as *aniseikonia*, that is abnormal unequal monocular perceptual images.

In equality of image was taken as a problem in producing defective binocular vision and defective spatial localization in the past also. Minus and plus spherical and cylindrical lenses effect on ocular images. They were of the opinion that there effects are produced in cases of anisometropia and could be eliminated by the constant use of glasses. Size of the retinal image could be equalized with proper correction of anisometropia by placing the lenses 15 mm from the cornea.

It is generally believed that if equal images could be achieved there is relief in symptoms, but if uncorrected, it causes squint and amblyopia. Later it was observed that aniseikonia is independent of any refractive error as it was seen in emmetropia also but in large number of cases it was present with anisometropia and there was relief from symptoms after correction with iseikonic lenses. Aniseikonia causes no trouble in congenital or in developmental cases, "but disturbances may develop when the refraction is corrected in adults.

CAUSES OF ANISEIKONIA

Aniseikonia can be due to optical, anatomical or central causes.

Optical Causes

Aniseikonia is most commonly due to anisometropia. The basic images and the corrected images vary in size according to whether the basic images are axial or refractive, whether they are corrected with minus or plus lenses. In axial refractive error there is increase or decrease in image size by 2% for every diopter in hypermetropia and myopia respectively, whereas in refractive aniseikonia there is increase or decrease in size of the image of about 0.5% per diopter.

Anatomical Causes

Neuroanatomy of retinal receptor mechanism (Rods and cones) effects the retinal images. If the cones are crowded the image will be shortened and if they are separated it will be larges. If also depends on distribution of neural receptors in retina. Aniseikonia may be found in patients after detachment operation, macular lesions and certain corneal scars.

Central Causes

In cases of emmetropia, aniseikonia may be present which suggests that aniseikonia is not always the result of anisometropia but probably the brain perceives asymmetrically in these cases. Thus it also depends on certain psychological factors of the perspective mechanism especially with simultaneous perception and with previous perceptual habits and knowledge. In such cases either patient is having low threshold or hypersensitivity.

Physical factors like asymmetric convergence, physical character of the object like size, shape, position and distance of the object also affects the retinal images.

CLASSIFICATION OF ANISEIKONIA

Aniseikonia may be physiological and abnormal or anomalous.

Physiological Aniseikonia

A slight difference in size and shape of the retinal images of the two eyes occurs normally and this retinal disparity is because of lateral separation of the eyes and is responsible for stereoscopic interpretation of space. This discrepancy is compensated psychologically and does not give rise to symptoms. Aniseikonia can be produced in two normal eyes by attending the luminance of an object presented to one of the eyes on the two equal objects the brighter will appear to be larger.

Abnormal or Anomalous Aniseikonia

Etiologically it may be:

Optical

When aniseikonia is because of optical phenomenon, known as optical abnormal aniseikonia. It may be:

a. *Inherent:* It depends on difference in dioptric system of the two eyes, e.g. anisometropia.
b. *Acquired:* It depends on the correcting lenses worn, their power position, thickness and form.

Anatomical

It depends upon the density of the retinal mosaic, i.e. distribution of rods and cones, and perhaps other factors at the perceptual level concerned with the simultaneous perception of the two visual images, a matter about which little is known. Aniseikonia is classified as:

i. *Normal physiological aniseikonia*: As described by Duke Elder (1970)
ii. *Abnormal aniseikonia*: He proposed the following classification to abnormal aniseikonia depending upon the axis in which aniseikonia exists.
   a. Meridional axis 180°
   b. Meridional axis 90°
   c. Overall
   d. Cyclo type due to oblique cylinders
   e. Asymmetric type.

According to another school of thought aniseikonia may be classified as:

i. *Physiological or normal:* As described by Duke Elder (1970)
ii. *Inherent:* Which exists with emmetropia or isometropia and can be considered as anatomic congenital or inherent type
iii. *Induced:* This type of aniseikonia which is induced by the correction of anisometropia and also that type of aniseikonia which is induced by changes in base curve or thickness, or by distance of the lens from eye.

The image size of difference in image sizes are overall symmetrical or meridional, the retinal image of one eye is symmetrically longer or smaller in one meridian than of the other or the retinal image of one eye is symmetrically larger in one meridian than that of the other or the retinal image of one eye is symmetrically larger in one meridian and smaller in another than that of the other eye.

Asymmetrical when there is difference in shape.

a. A progressive increase or decrease in size across the visual axis with plus or minus lenses.
b. Irregular distortion of the image or the combination of above.

Easy and comfortable fusion of the two retinal images demands that there is as equal as possible in brightness, from and size when an aniseikonia is present but as the last requirement is not fulfilled aniseikonia, therefore, is an obstacle to fusion. If the centers of the images are fused, the peripheral margins are not and *vice versa*. However, central fusion is mostly commonly affected in aniseikonia due to predominance of fovea in binocular vision. If the aniseikonia is very small, the difficulty is negligible, but it is large say 4.5% or more, the patient will suppress part of the image of one eye, making fusion difficult, or suppression, amblyopia and deviation may supervene. There is a tremendous controversy on tolerance of aniseikonia. It is generally believed that 5% aniseikonia is physiological while even 20% may be tolerated, while even 3% may produce symptoms. There is variance in tolerance in aniseikonia by individual patients.

Aniseikonia also affects localization depending upon if the aniseikonia is horizontal or vertical or both, effect on stereopsis may also occur. However, these may disappear. When the patient is adjusted to the correction a, conversation occur physiologically, through the aniseikonia basically may remain the same.

OPTICS

Spectacle Magnification

It is defined as the ratio of the retinal image size in the corrected ametropic eye to that in the uncorrected eye, having reference to an object at infinity. The spectacle magnification is always greater than unity for a convex lens and less than unity for a concave lens. A concept that a correcting lens placed at the anterior focal point of an eye does not alter the size of the retinal image is also a misconception.

Magnification with Contact Lenses

As the correcting lens approach the eye, the magnification approaches unity. This, of courses, is the case when considering a contact lens. The contact lens greatly affects the size of the image. The retinal image size is greater or lesser than unity in hypermetropia and myopia respectively, when corrected with glasses. Since contact lens are worn in contact with the cornea, they reduce the retinal image size in hypermetropia and increase it in myopia in comparison with the glasses.

MEASUREMENT OF ANISEIKONIA

Various methods of measuring aniseikonia are described from time to time which, are as follows:

Clinical Instrument

A clinical instrument for the measurement of aniseikonia was essentially a heploscope and is original eikonometer of Amas. The principle of the instrument was simply by presenting two images, one to each eye, in a reflecting stereoscopes. Fusion was prevented by employing dissimilar objects of the same size of such a design the discrepancies between them could not be readily assessed. The magnitude of difference in size of the ocular images is determined by employing a series of 'C' power lenses that magnify the size of image.

Horopter Apparatus

The principle of this apparatus the same as above. There are similar objects in the field of view which fuse and dissimilar object determinable lateral distances which do not fuse. It differ, however, in that the similar objects are at the point of fixation, while the dissimilar are images on peripheral retina and the position of the dissimilar objects can varied laterally to each other. Patient maintaining his fixation coincides the each line with solid lines by moving the handle. The position of wire gives the distance of corresponding retinal points from fixation point at the particular peripheral angle. Many peripheral angles are taken and image disparity in horizontal meridian is determined.

Standard Eikonometer

The target used is composed of four pairs of lines arranged round a central fixation mark. The central fixation mark is seen by both eyes, the light from the even number line is polarized in one direction and the light from the odd number line is polarized to other direction through polarizing filter. Any abnormality in conceding the lines will reveal the aniseikonia. Meridional aniseikonia can also be measured.

Space Eikonometer

The best technique so far devised is of space eikonometer. This is based upon the fact that when the incongruity of the ocular image differs from normal, anomalous spatial localization must necessarily result. If spatial localization is removed from accessory aids and uniocular clues and the patient has to rely solely upon desparities of the image of the two eyes. Any image desparity is measured by neutralizing the displacement of image with iseikonic lenses. The sensitivity of the instrument is up to 0.05 percent of the image desparity.

Maddox Rod Test

Two Maddox rods were placed before the two eyes to obtain a binocular image of two vertical streaks from two muscle lights, the streaks will appear at unequal distances from the observer if aniseikonia is present at the axis of 90°. If aniseikonia is at 180° then three lights will appear, on in center of each line. Thus, aniseikonia in horizontal meridian can be known space eikonometer is the most satisfactory technique. Here target slides for amblyoscope bases on Ames vertical and cross with the subject fusing the two slides while the arms of synaptophore are slowly diverged about 0.250 at each interval. At certain point the image will break as the lines on the side of the eye receiving larger image will occur as fusion break. This should be repeated for confirmation. In front of the eye receiving small image as determined as 5% aniseikonic lens is placed and the test is repeated, if the result is revised then the 5% lens is reduced gradually untill a neutral point is reached, when the breaking of the lines occur at the same time and to the same amount on each slide. To measure aniseikonia over 5% to axis 1.05 slide is used with 5% lens and test is repeated.

Aniseikonia

Symptoms are both subjective and visual. Patients with difference in image size may feel visual symptoms as well as asthenopic symptoms. Aniseikonis interferes with the smooth functioning of visual discomfort, eye stain, burning, itching, blurred vision, diplopia fixation difficulty and squint. Fusion mechanism demands adjustment of visual axes of the two eyes so that images, fall, not on exactly corresponding point but on non-corresponding areas thus eyes are whipped up to accurate focusing fixation and fusion.

Patients may develop neurotic symptoms like tenseness, irritability, vertigo, headache and exhaustion. Patient may be having gastric disturbance like gastritis, nausea, vomiting and indigestion are also associated symptoms in aniseikonic patients.

Large number of cases show a partial and local suppression which takes place only at fovea, patient often feels slanting of the surface and ups and down on waling aniseikonia and may be compensated after the use of glasses.

Small differences in size of the retinal image of the two eyes are not generally appreciated and it is likely that these do not impair binocular vision. As a general rule differences upto 5% can be compensated by the plasticity of visual perceptive mechanism but such compensation may impair the effectiveness of depth perception. Stereopsia markedly improves after correction of such disparity when the difference is in excess of this and or compensatory power is poor binocular vision becomes difficult or been impossible. Suppression and amblyopia may develop at an early stage in such cases. If however, binocular vision has already been well-established and sudden marked aniseikonia may be introduced (as in monocular aphakia) diplopia and other consequences may develop which have to be appropriately dealt with tolerance to aniseikonia can also be helpful in maintaining the binocular vision and preventing amblyopia.

Abnormal difference between the size and/or shape of the ocular images in a horizontal direction deranges the apparent position of objects in visual field. This causes an apparent horizontal rotation of the visual field and may affect the fusion process. There much as fusion because in general depth perception from the disparity of images in each eyes.

In higher degrees, aniseikonia causes imperfect binocular vision, but in lower degrees in earlier life it causes eye strain. It was accordingly observed in the investigation on aniseikonia and fusion that large majority of cases with convergence insufficiency had poor tolerance to aniseikonia and those with better fusion had better tolerance. Gradually increasing aniseikonia steudily reduced fusion range and affected fusion ultimately.

MANAGEMENT

Small degree of aniseikonia may be corrected by iseikonic lenses. These lenses cause magnification without introducing appreciable refractive power by changing the beam of rays passing through them. Magnification in one or in all meridian can be given in iseikonic lenses to suit the regular aniseikonia.

The fact that as we approaches the modal point of the eye, the magnification approaches unity, prompted the idea of contact lenses. Contact lenses reduce aniseikonia considerably and binocular function can also improve with contact lenses.

Aniseikonia is disturbing in monocular saphakia even with contact lenses though binocular functions are fairly good residual aniseikonia has been affectively reduced by the prescription of a combination of over powered contact lens and minus spectacle glass. It is tolerated well and improves the binocular function and therefore prevents onset of amblyopia.

18 Nystagmus

Rhythmic rapidity to and fro movement of the eyes is called *nystagmus*. Type of nystagmus described based one certain characteristics like rate (rapid or slow), amplitue (corse or fine), direction (horizontal, vertical or rotational), and type of movements (pendular or jerky). Nystagmus is pendular where eye movements in each direction are equal. On the other hand it is called jerky when there is slow component in one direction and fact component in opposite direction.

SPECIFIC TYPES

I. *Congenital*: It is usually present at birth but may be noticed by parents within a few months. Most commonly it is a horizontal nystagmus. Acromatopia and hypophasia of the optic nerve may be present. Usually the nystagmus reduced is of totally absent in a certain direction of gaze the patient's null point. Visual acuity is best tested at null point.

   Latent nystagmus is type of congenital jerk nystagmus appearing on attempted fixation, when other eye is covered. Rapid irregular random eye movement in all direction of gaze are seen in cases of laber's congenital amaurosis or hypoplastic optic nerve. Head nodding and head taking is seen more frequently in congenital that acquired nystagmus.

   Spasmus nutans is a condition featuring nystagmus, head nodding and toticallie with onset between the age of 4 to 12 months.

II. *Down beating nystagmus*: When fast phase of nystagmus is downwards.

III. *Up-beating nystagmus*: When fast phase of nystagmus is upwards. This is a pattern of ocular movements in which the one eye elevates while the other depresses, usually accompanied by intorsion and extorsion on elevation and depression respectively.

IV. *Periodic alternating nystagmus*: It is jerky type of nystagmus which shows rhythmic change in direction and amplitude.

V. *Physiological nystagmus*: There 2 forms of phenomenon-optokine nystagmus and caloric nystagmus. Optokinetic nystagmus result when a person gazed at a succession of object-moving fast in one direction for example, looking at the outside object, through a window of a fast moving train-rail road nystagmus. The eyes follow one object slowly and then return quickly to fixate at the next object. When warm or water is irrigated in the external auditory canal, convention correct are produced in the semicircular canal resulting in calonic nystagmus.

In cold water irrigation the induced has a fast phase in the direction opposite ear. If warm is used the fact phase will be on the same side.

Index

A

B

C

D

E

F

G

H

L

M

N

O

P

R

S

T

V

W